A Dancer's Diary

A comprehensive guide to everything a dancer needs to know for staying healthy and strong throughout the year

By

AMANDA E. HOWARD

Forward by

CAROL PERKINS N.D.

Illustrations by

JULIA HOWARD

Photography and Cover by

STEPHEN HOWARD

Dedication and Acknowledgments

First, I want to thank my Heavenly Father for all He has blessed me with. I have been blessed with so many experiences and opportunities. I truly believe that He has a plan for my life bigger and better than anything I could ever hope or imagine!

To my Mom who, thanks to my wonderful Grandma who taught her everything she knows, taught me everything I know. Thanks for teaching me to love learning new things and to share my love of learning with others. And thank you for being my support in hard times, and for the many words of wisdom you have supplied over the years.

To my Dad for teaching me all about business and for helping me start up one of my own. I could not have done it without you! Thank you for being my personal editor and for putting up with all my questions. I also want to thank you for the beautiful job you did with all the photography! You are pretty awesome.

Grandma, thank you for your help in creating this book. I am so blessed to have you!

Thanks to my entire family for supporting me in all my endeavors, big and small. I know I have had big ideas and you have all helped me to achieve them. You are an awesome family and I thank God every day for the blessings and love you have supplied! I love you all very much.

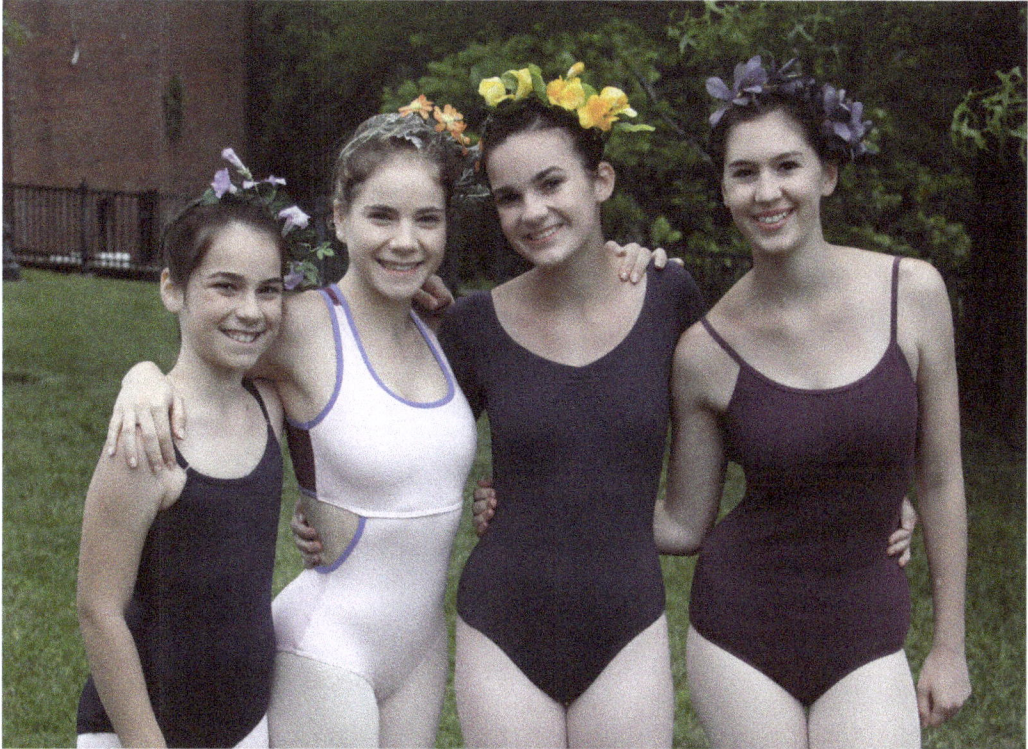

I also want to thank Ryley, Ava, Julia, and Riley for being my beautiful models. I loved working with you girls and I hope to work with you again in the future. Working with you was one of the highlights of putting *A Dancer's Diary* together and I couldn't have done it without you!

CONTENTS

PART TWO

Healthy Dancer

PART THREE

Happy Dancer

PART FOUR

Beautiful Dancer

PART FIVE

Fun Stuff

Introduction

WHAT TO EXPECT

Are you a dancer looking for new ways to maintain a healthy lifestyle? Are you a dance instructor looking for ways to teach your students how to care for their bodies? Are you struggling to find a resource that has all the information you need in one condensed publication?

Whether you are an up and coming ballerina or an involved dance instructor, this book will outline all the information you need to maintain a healthy and active lifestyle.

- You will discover how to effectively achieve your truest potential as a dancer by unlocking the secrets to flexibility
- Take care of and prevent various common dance injuries
- Learn how to make your own at-home "spa" products
- Achieve the ability to stay calm under pressure
- Learn how to menu plan based on your personal dietary needs
- Maintain a strong immune system even during the coldest months
- And how to maintain a healthy weight.

I wrote this book so that instructors and dancers of all ages could have one valuable resource of information that they could consistently go back to. Years of research and collaborations has brought this scientifically proven, doctor recommended, dancer tested information. My goal is for dancers, as well as instructors, to become more educated in health and wellness focused on an active lifestyle.

You will also have the opportunity to learn some anatomy and basic function of your body. Charts and illustrations are carefully created to help you understand what you read. Everything is written in an easily accessible and understandable way in order to avoid confusion, and is always backed up by sufficient evidence.

Now that you understand what to expect, let's get started!

Forward

By Carol Perkins, N.D.

I am blessed to know Amanda Howard, not only because she is my granddaughter, but because she is one of the most committed, insightful, and knowledgeable persons that I know. Our mutual reverence for God and our quest to seek timeless health truths have made us "kindred spirits" on a mission that is beyond even the scope of our imagination. Always willing to step outside the proverbial "box," Amanda is constantly looking for ways to refine and improve her skills and protocols.

As a naturopathic doctor for the past 17 years in Lexington, Kentucky, one of my greatest passions is to help people reach their highest life potential. My goal with each patient is to identify the *root cause* of their illness and then design the best protocol to restore them to optimal health. Amanda's holistic approach in her book, *A Dancer's Diary*, is very similar – she addresses not only the body, but also the mind and spirit.

Amanda has used her love of dance to teach young dancers how to use it to glorify God and inspire others. For two years, she owned a dance studio, Praise Him with a Dance, until she decided that she wanted to expand her horizons. Recently Amanda has become a certified Personal Fitness Trainer and Health Specialist. Her dream is to teach others how to stay healthy and strong in order to achieve their highest potentials.

There are many books written about dancing - some address dance techniques while others give tips about weight control and nutrition. But *A Dancer's Diary* is the most comprehensive guide to a dancer's needs that I have found.

As a naturopathic doctor, I teach the importance of **PREVENTION** to my patients. So I am very impressed that Amanda includes many techniques for prevention of injuries as well as what to do if one gets an injury.

Equally important in prevention is a healthy diet and lifestyle. Amanda has learned first-hand how to shop wisely, cook delicious meals and eat to stay well. She gives menu planning tips, snack ideas, foods to avoid, when to eat, how to stay hydrated and some great-tasting recipes.

I absolutely love Chapter Ten – Taking Care of Your Dancing Feet, Chapter Eleven – Healthy Hair and Chapter Twelve – Beauty Is More Than Skin Deep! You don't have to be a dancer to appreciate the valuable information contained in these chapters. She even includes wonderful recipes for making your own homemade beauty products!

These are just a few of the health secretes you will learn from reading and using this book. *A Dancer's Diary* is not a book to read once and put on your shelf to collect dust; instead, certainly for the recipes but also for the health and dietary insight, you'll find yourself referring back to it often as your trusted "guide to everything a dancer needs to know for staying healthy and strong throughout the year."

Disclaimer

In this book, I have suggested many nutritional strategies and supplements that can aid you in your health. These suggestions are written to inform the interested reader of options related to health and fitness. I hope to provide you with information that can act as a nutritional guide and not a diagnosis or treatment.

All the information you will read is based on up-to-date information and has been found through extensive research. None of the suggestions related to supplements are meant to treat or cure any disease. Any information that you find on illness and injury are not meant to replace your doctor. If you have a severe injury or are extremely ill, please see you doctor immediately.

Everything regarding health can be changed based on the individual and may not work the same for everyone. I have provided special journal pages that you can fill out according to your own individual needs and what works for you.

Please use this book as an educational source. See a nutritional specialist if you need further assistance in building a meal plan based on your body type and any health needs. All product recommendations can be found in the back of the book. Please run any new supplements by your doctor before taking them.

Glamorous Dancers of the Silver Screen

I have always had a fascination with old movies—the way men acted like gentlemen and the women were always ladies. My favorite type of old movies, are the musicals. They always make me feel happy and light-hearted. The singing is romantic and sometimes silly, and the dancing—oh the wonderful dancing! That is my favorite part. Each star has their own style and they perform it flawlessly. This is why I watch these movies!

Movie musicals reached their height of fame during the first half of the 20th century and we found captivating new dance icons that blew us away—Fred Astaire, Gene Kelly, Ginger Rogers, Cyd Charisse, Mitzi Gaynor, Judy Garland, and Leslie Caron to name a few. They made the dancing look effortless and looked as if they were floating. These dancers were the pioneers who set the stage for Hollywood's dance-film genre with famous routines such as *Singin' in the Rain* (Kelly), *Cheek to Cheek* (Astaire), and *We're off to see the Wizard* (Garland). These fabulous dancers danced to have fun and used it as a way to inspire creativity in others. They made even the un-coordinated and "2 left feet" folks want to get up and dance, too.

We will always remember Fred Astaire dancing on the walls and ceiling in *Royal Wedding*, Audrey Hepburn doing her crazy contemporary dance in *Funny Face*, the frontier guys dancing to impress the girls in *Seven Brides for Seven Brothers*, Donald O'Connor flipping off the walls in *Make 'Em Laugh*, Dick Van Dyke and Julie Andrews in *Mary Poppins*, and of course Gene Kelly soaked through while "singin' and dancing in the rain."

Fred Astaire is sometimes characterized as Mr. Elegance. He was delicate and graceful but powerful. Every time he danced, there was a story attached, full of emotion. Gene Kelly was strong and athletic. He could lift a lady and dance with her in his arms as if she were nothing but a feather. Let us also not forget his signature move, the airplane. In *An American in Paris* we see him do twelve or more in succession!

The women of the screen were beautiful and poised. Ginger Rogers was at her best alongside Fred Astaire, making them one of the most famous dancing couples. Her ballroom dancing was graceful and her tap, fun and exciting. The we see Judy Garland. Her voice and dance moves could never be equaled. There are no words to describe how incredible she was! Her dancing was energetic and so much fun to watch.

Inspiring and oh, so unforgettable! We are thankful that they left behind their wonderful movies for us to enjoy.

I wanted to share my love for these people and their movies because I want to encourage you dancers out there to be inspiring. To encourage others to find joy and creativity in dance through your movements and expressions. I encourage you to tell a story with your dance and to have fun with it. Sometimes as ballerinas, we tend to be too serious. We need to let loose and just have some fun on occasion. Our role is to inspire and give back to others using our talents.

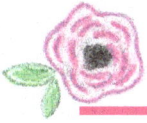

"Always be a first-rate version of yourself, instead of a second-rate version of somebody else."
    –Judy Garland

"The finest all-around performer we ever had in America was Judy Garland. There was no limit to her talent. She was the quickest, brightest person I ever worked with."
    –Gene Kelly

"You know, that Kelly, he's just terrific. That's all there is to it. He dances like crazy, he directs like crazy. I adore this guy. I really am crazy about his work."
    –Fred Astaire

"I suppose I made it look easy, but gee whiz, did I work and worry."
    –Fred Astaire

"The most important thing in anyone's life is to be giving something. The quality I can give is fun, joy and happiness. This is my gift."
    –Ginger Rogers

"I adore the man. I always have adored him. It was the most fortunate thing that ever happened to me, being teamed with Fred: he was everything a little starry-eyed girl from a small town ever dreamed of."
    –Ginger Rogers

"I never wanted to be a dancer. It's true! I wanted to be a shortstop for the Pittsburgh Pirates."
    –Gene Kelly

"Fred could never do the lifts Gene did and never wanted to. I'd say they were the two greatest dancing personalities who were ever on the screen. Each has a distinctive style. Each is a joy to work with. But it's like comparing apples and oranges. They're both delicious."
    –Cyd Charisse

"If I had to give up either acting or dancing, I'd choose to keep dancing."
    –Cyd Charisse

"Dancing is still the hardest profession. Gene Kelly said dancing is a man's game. Women have to do the same thing in heels, and have to sing and smile at the same time. Professional athletes don't even have to do that – and they get to wear sneakers."
    –Mitzi Gaynor

A Brief History of Dance

Dance has always been a part of society as a form of ceremony, ritual, celebration, worship, and entertainment. The Greeks around 600 B.C. used dance as a form of worship to their god, Dionysus. Archeologists have found many drawings in old Egyptian and Indian tombs that depict human figures dancing.

The term "ballet" came from the Italian word *"ballare"* which means to dance. Ballet was originally founded in the Italian Renaissance courts during the early part of the 15th century. Dance masters would teach the nobility various steps that would become elaborate performances for weddings, balls, and other celebrations. The very first steps included small hops, slides, curtsies, promenades, and turns. What we know today as ballroom or social dance is what started the contemporary dance history.

Catherine de Medici, wife of King Henry II of France, loved the arts and began to fund ballet performances. This led to the formation of *ballet de cour*, programs that included dance, costumes, music, décor, and poetry. Over the next hundred years or so, the French established the official dance terminology and vocabulary. During the 17th century, King Louis XIV popularized this art form because of his love of dance, as he was a performer himself.

The court dances grew until they were moved to elevated platforms so that a larger audience to attend the elaborate performances. The first dance academy was opened in 1661 in Paris. The French opera *Le Triomphe de l'Amour* became a long-standing tradition in France as it incorporated ballet alongside the opera performance. French ballet master, Jean Georges Noverre believed that ballet could stand on its own and created performances that introduced *ballet d'action*, a style of dance that was used to tell a story.

Classical ballet became a well-known art form during the first half of the 19th century with dances like *Giselle* and *La Sylphide*. Pointe work also became the norm during this period as well as the tutu.

Russia took ballet to new heights by creating the popular ballets, *The Nutcracker*, *The Sleeping Beauty*, and *Swan Lake*. They became the leading creative center for the dance world. Russian choreographers wanted to create ballet performances that displayed classical technique, precision of movement, proper turnout and extension, as well as pointe work. The shorter tutu was also introduced to show the difficult movements the dancer was performing.

In the early twentieth century, the Ballet Russes was formed by Serge Diaghilev. They toured Europe and America presenting a wide variety of ballets. It was not until 1930 that ballet started to develop as a popular form of dance in America due to the settlement of several of Diaghilev's dancers, the most popular being George Balanchine.

George Balanchine changed ballet even more with his contemporary ideas. His ballets had no story to tell and were simply to show human emotion and power. Most choreographers during the 20th century saw ballet as being too restrictive and "old-fashioned." As a result, choreographers such as Martha Graham and Merce Cunningham used the foundations of ballet to create a whole new style of dance—contemporary. This allowed for creative growth and expression.

Throughout the years, ballet has inspired many different styles of dance including tap, jazz, hip-hop, and contemporary. Choreographers and dancers continue to come up with new ideas that push the boundaries of traditional dance forms. They are creating new ways to express human emotion and tell stories.

"Today's appreciation of ballet continues to grow as more people learn the complexities of the dance and view the art form. Knowing the history of ballet frames the dance through its importance throughout time." **–LuAnn Schindler**

PART ONE

Strong Dancer

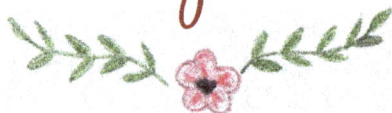

CHAPTER ONE

Cross Training and Conditioning

---

*"In dance, fatigue is a factor in 90% of injuries and overuse contributes to 65% of dance injuries. Fatigue and overuse injuries can become chronic problems that trouble the dancer daily. Cross training **and conditioning** can help reduce risk of these types of injuries by balancing out the muscles and the body and providing relief to the muscles that are constantly worked." **–Leigh Heflin** (MSc Dance Science) [emphasis added]*

THE IMPORTANCE OF CROSS TRAINING

Ballet focuses on strength, control, and flexibility and only works certain areas of the body, leaving any unused muscles to weaken over time. Dancers should train in other areas such as swimming, fast walking, or cycling to strengthen other muscle groups and promote cardiovascular health. It is also great to take different styles of dance to gain a wider range of experience as well as to strengthen technique. If you take ballet, think about taking other classes such as tap, jazz, or contemporary.

Keeping your workout balanced is key to creating a proper schedule. If you are in the studio 4-5 days out of the week, you might want to try supplementing your routine with release exercises that do not build up more tension (i.e. Pilates and flexibility training). If you are only dancing for 2-3 days out of the week, you might want to try supplementing your routine with workouts that focus on strengthening different areas of your body and get your heart pumping (i.e. cardio and TABATA).

In order to avoid over-exercising, it is best to attend dance class up to five times a week for only one hour rather than fitting in three classes per week for more than two hours. If this is unavoidable, do not add in any other exercise programs the rest of the week, instead do flexibility stretching.

It is important to be strong as well as flexible. Weight training is a great way to build strength and tone muscles. It can also help prevent overuse injuries due to over-flexibility. Use light weights to avoid gaining too much muscle mass. I recommend 3-5 pound weights.

Dancers should try to avoid running and jogging as much as possible because of the constant pounding on the joints and delicate bones in the feet and ankles. It can also put pressure on your Achilles tendon and knees due to the turn-out of the feet and legs. I recommend fast walking as a substitute.

Pilates promotes flexibility and balance and is very relaxing to the muscles, which makes it a great choice for dancers who need a break during the week. Try using some of the flexibility exercises that we talk about in chapter 3 for low impact exercising or take a Pilates class through your studio.

TABATA workouts are great for dancers and other athletes who need to build up their cardio and strength. I recommend these workouts for dancers who are only going to the studio 2-3 times a week because they are high impact and very effective. The idea behind TABATA is to train rigorously for twenty seconds with a rest of ten seconds in between, totaling eight repetitions per exercise.

Another great way to increase circulation and promote cardiovascular health is by jumping on a trampoline. Jumping promotes lymph drainage by using gravity to increase lymph flow without stressing the body. Try a trampoline workout sometime and have fun with it.

Make sure that you are not over-exercising during the week as this can lead to exercise-induced health issues and injury. You should only workout a couple of times per week, in addition to ballet, depending on your age and weight. Try to stick to exercising for only 15-20 minutes a day in addition to your dance training. Adults and adolescents should not do more than 25-30 minutes of aerobic exercise per day. Strength training should take up at least 15-20 minutes of their exercise time as well.

THE IMPORTANCE OF CONDITIONING

It is important for dancers as well as other athletes to do conditioning exercises.

Conditioning exercises help reduce injury and raise athletic capabilities. Some examples of these type of exercises include calisthenics, plyometrics, weight training, and aerobic fitness. The purpose of conditioning is to gain muscle memory by performing specific movements based on athletic ability. The movements are repetitive and increase the amount of stress that the body can handle before an injury can occur, making the muscles more tolerant.

Calisthenics are exercises that use repetitive and rhythmical movements to gain strength, flexibility, and muscle memory. This type of exercise uses a lot of your own bodyweight instead of equipment and is performed in 15-20 repetitions of each exercise (i.e. push-ups, squats, burpees, mountain climbers, etc.).

Plyometrics is a great type of exercise for gaining strength in the legs and glutes. These exercises include a lot of jumping and hopping performed in repetitions of 20-30 (i.e. jumping jacks, squat jumps, etc.).

A strong core is important to take the pressure off the lower back and support the rest of the body while balancing. One of the best ways to keep your core strong is by performing planks. I have provided a regular version and a modified version of both a regular plank and a side plank.

Try and hold each plank for 60-90 seconds, keeping your abs tight, butt tucked under, and neck long.

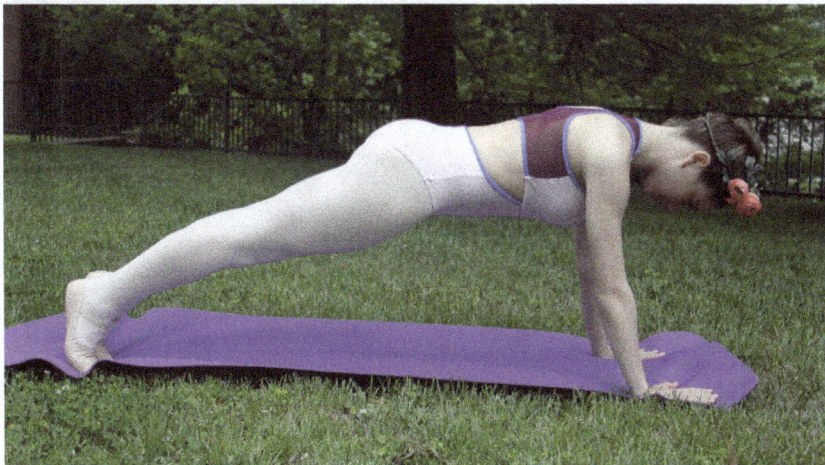

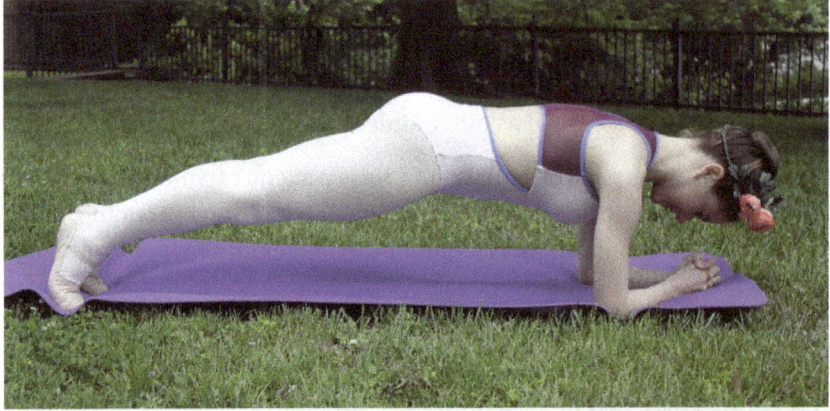

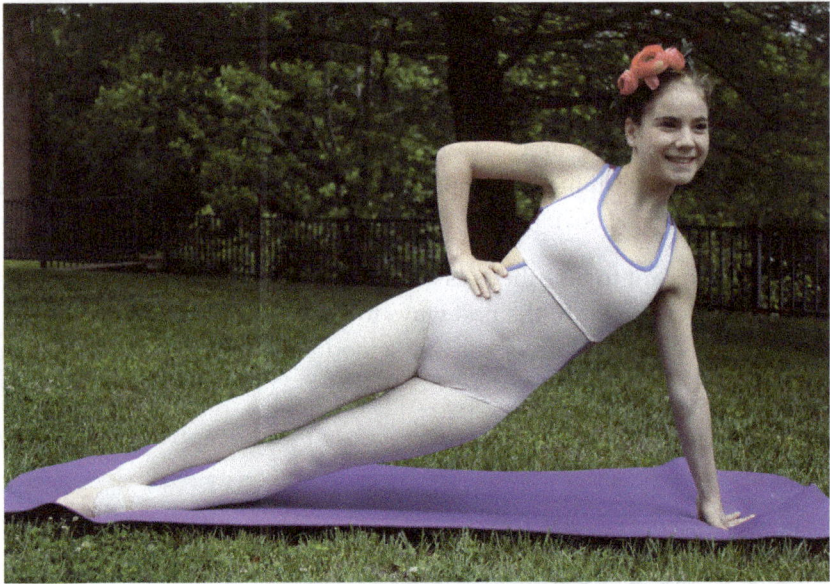

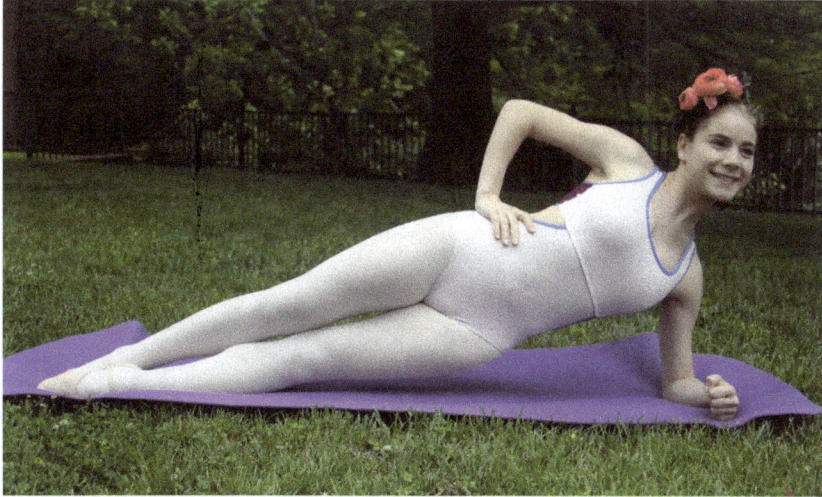

You can also perform low crunches, bicycle crunches, and crunches on an exercise ball to build up abdominal strength. Repeat each exercise at least 20 times.

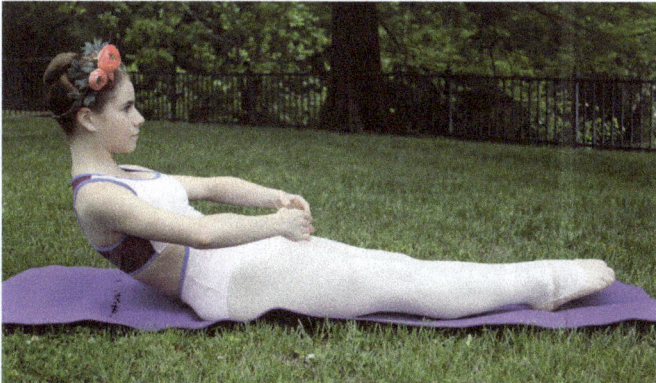

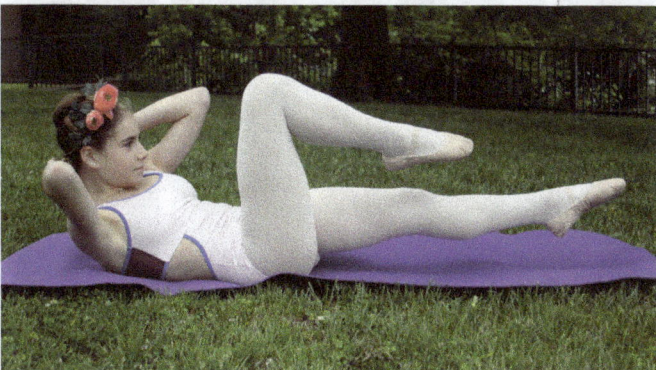

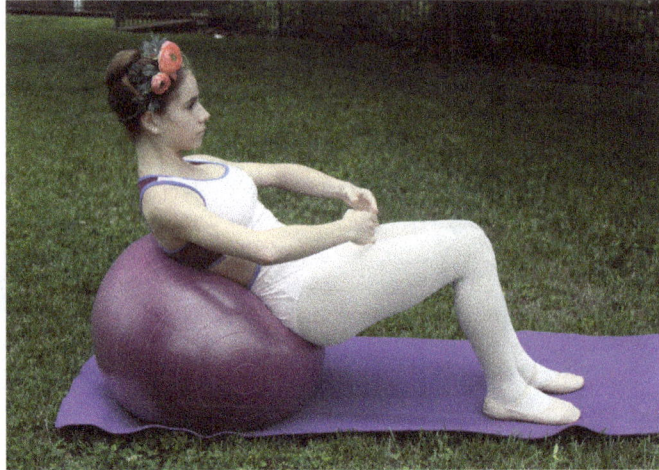

Strong arms are important especially when you are in dance. Holding positions for long periods of time can be exhausting. Try doing graceful ballet-like movements with your arms and small, controlled circles. You can also do low triceps extensions by keeping your hands behind your hips and using only the weight of your arms.

Float your arms up and down 20-30 times. Try to make circles high and low. Push your arms back behind your hips. You would not think that these exercises would work, but they are suprisingly effective.

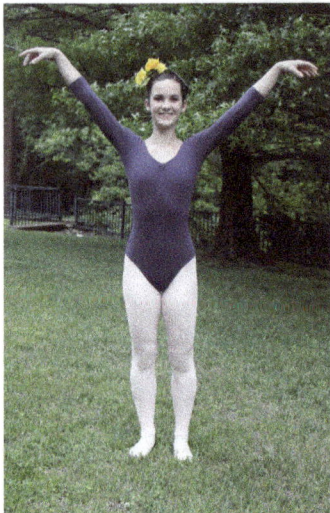

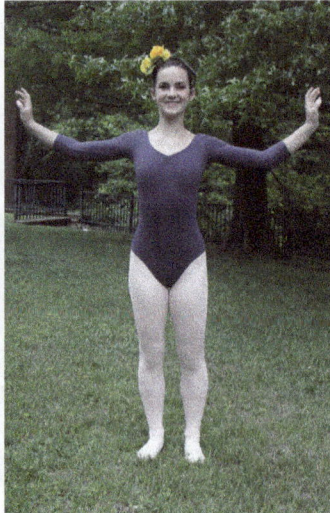

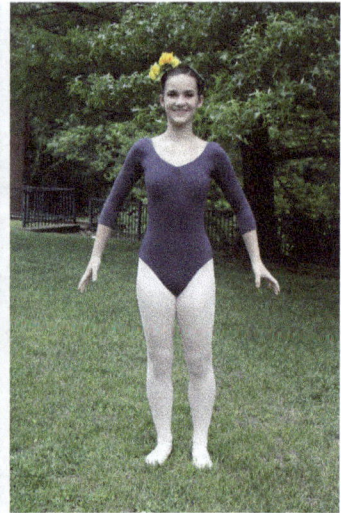

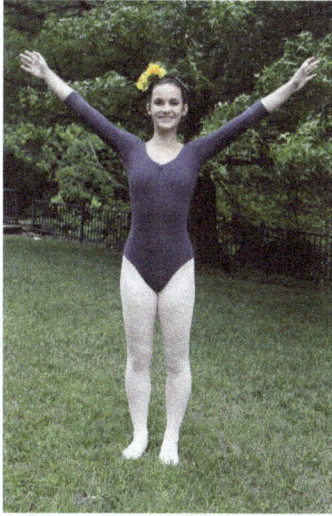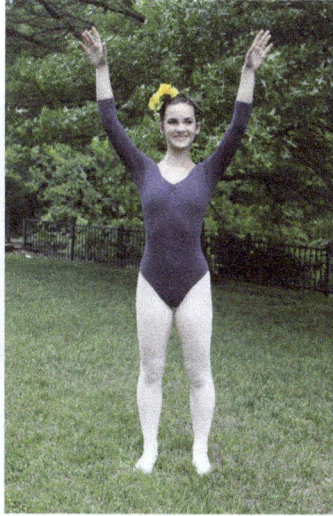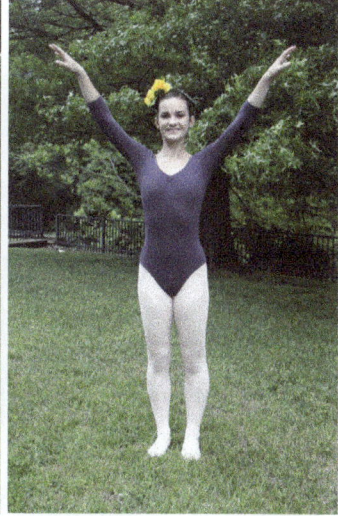
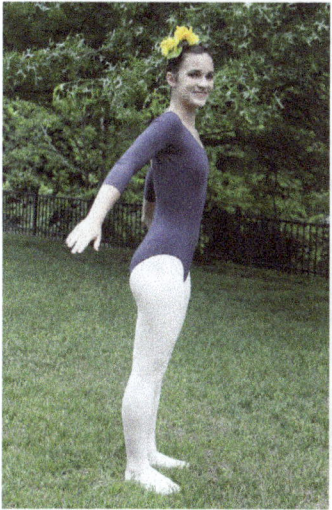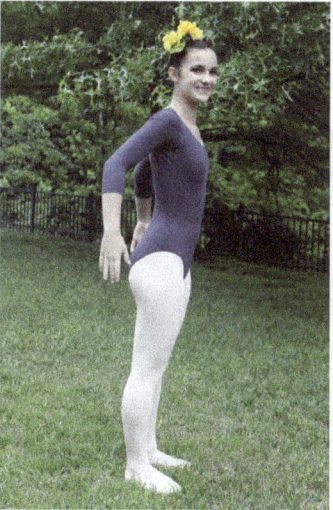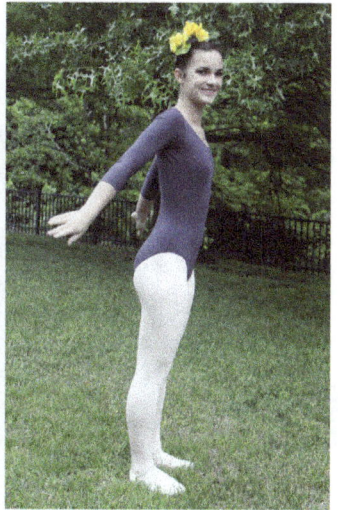

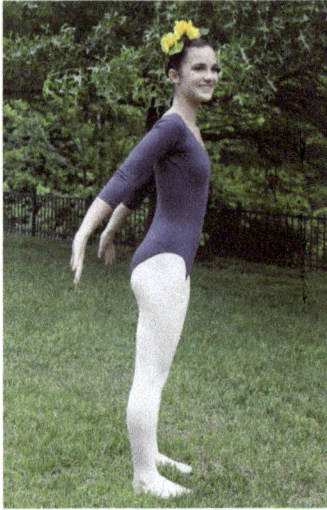

You can also try seated rows to exercise the back of the arms, using a TheraBand. Make sure your back is straight and stationary the whole time. Repeat the exercise 10-20 times.

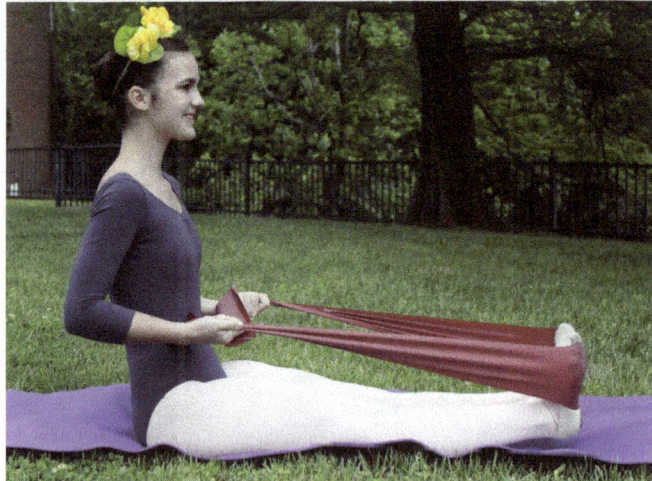

To strengthen your ankles and feet, elastic training is great.

Wrap a TheraBand around your foot and pointe and flex 20-30 times. Hold the band in front of you, keeping it taught.

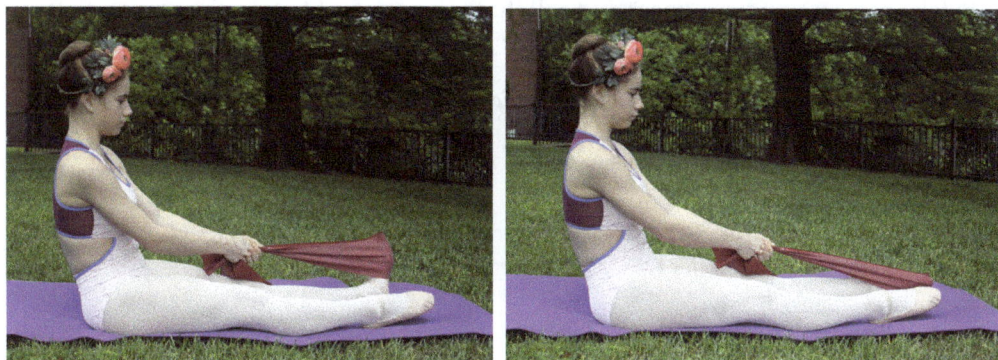

AEROBIC VS. ANAEROBIC FITNESS

Aerobic

Aerobic fitness is most commonly known as "cardio." Aerobic exercises stimulate and strengthen the heart in order to improve its pumping efficiency. They also activate your immune system and elevate your mood by the increase of endorphins.

Most aerobic exercises are low intensity and are performed for longer periods of time. Walking, interval running, rowing, cycling, hiking, dancing, cross-country skiing, swimming, fast walking, and kickboxing are some great examples of fun aerobic exercises.

Swimming is great for increasing aerobic capacity and strengthens the mid and upper body muscles. Studies have found that walking in the water can reduce lower back pain. It is also great for stress reduction. Swimming allows your muscles and joints to relax and float, washing away stress and tension. The resistance of the water helps tone muscles and the regulated breathing patterns help you take in more oxygen. It is good to try different strokes to work on different parts of your body. Try alternating between breaststroke, backstroke, and freestyle.

Running can be very hard on a dancer's joints and ligaments so I do not usually recommend it. However, if you do choose to run, try performing intervals. Fast walk for ten minutes and run for ten minutes. Make sure you wear supportive running shoes to support your Achilles, ankles, and arches. While you are running, make sure you are engaging all your leg muscles to prevent over exercising of one area. Use your thighs and hips to take pressure off your knees and roll through your foot to take the pressure off your feet and ankles.

Aerobic fitness has many benefits, some of which include:
- *The increase of oxygen in the body*
- *Improved circulation*
- *Lower blood pressure*
- *Increase in red blood cell count making the transport of oxygen more efficient*
- *Improved mental health*
- *Lower stress levels*
- *Reduced risk of depression and diabetes*
- *Increase in blood flow to the muscles*
- *Enhanced recovery time*
- *Increased blood oxygen levels*
- *Increased endurance*
- *Increased ability to detoxify*

Anaerobic

Anaerobic fitness is more intense than aerobic and is typically used to increase muscle mass, endurance, and performance. It is usually performed with short bursts of energy for a short period of time. Due to the lack of oxygen being taken in, lactic acid tends to build up in the muscles faster. This can cause a slight burning feeling in the muscles and results in muscle fatigue, so make sure that you do less repetitions than you think you should.

Some anaerobic exercises include, isotonic, isometric, calisthenics, and sprinting. Isotonic exercises require weights to increase muscle strength. Isometric exercises are held for long periods of time to increase muscular flexibility and to strengthen the muscles (alpine skiing, mountain cycling, and wrestling).

To improve the body's endurance, callisthenic exercises are commonly used (squatting, push-ups, sit-ups, etc.). Finally, sprinting is most commonly used by athletes to increase overall metabolism. Sprinting tones and sculpts the muscles (marathon running), however I do not recommend this type of exercise for dancers.

If you choose to do anaerobic exercises, limit yourself to 20 minutes for only two times a week to prevent over-exercising. And stretch properly in between and after the exercises to prevent a buildup of lactic acid in the muscles.

EXERCISE INDUCED HEALTH ISSUES

All exercises can cause health problems if not properly monitored or performed.

Over-exercising is one of the most common issues dancers and other athletes must deal with. It is important to limit the amount of time that you exercise a day, making sure you fit in recovery time on the weekends. Exercising in the late afternoon or evening can cause insomnia so try and limit your exercising to the mornings and early afternoons.

Ways to prevent over-exercising:
- *Perform fewer repetitions*
- *Increase your recovery time*
- *Do not work out if you are feeling tired or you have no energy*
- *Do not exercise longer than thirty minutes a day*

If we exercise in excess, it is hard for our bodies to maintain homeostasis (the balance and maintenance of internal stability). Exercising up to an hour is acceptable but it is when you go over that hour that your body starts to stop benefitting from the exercise. In fact, exercising for 30 minutes a day is much more beneficial in the end than exercising for one hour.

When you exercise for more than an hour, your muscles will start to break down and you will become more susceptible to injury. It will also drain your adrenals making you more susceptible to illness and fatigue.

Microscopic tears occur in your muscles when you exercise. As they heal, your muscles get stronger. If you are exercising too much the tears will not heal properly and can lead to further injury. When doing anaerobic exercises, use lighter weights to prevent muscle strains and pulls, eat lots of protein and good fats after your workout to rebuild muscle, and drink plenty of water to keep yourself hydrated.

Too much cardio can cause overuse injuries and can also weaken your heart if performed too often. Limit your cardio routine to only twice a week for about 30 minutes.

If you ignore the signs of over-exercising it can put a strain on your liver and make it work harder to filter out the toxins in your blood. The body can go into anaerobic respiration, which is when too much lactic acid is created in your muscles. The liver is not able to keep up with the filtering process of lactic acid waste and in turn, will dump those toxins into the bloodstream.

Your body can also go into a catabolic state from the excess release of cortisol. This is when the body is put into a state of *alarm* and starts to attack your muscles. It starts to view your existing muscles as the enemy and stops creating new muscle. Your muscles start to break down and cause serious health issues such as Cushing's syndrome. Cushing's syndrome occurs when your body has been exposed to excess cortisol for long periods of time and can cause high blood pressure, bone loss, a rounded face, and sometimes diabetes.

Exercising increases endorphins that make you happy and have a lot of energy. Some people exercise just to give themselves this "energy high" and it can become very addicting. After a while, your body will start to break down and the "energy high" that you felt in the beginning will start to fade making you think you must do more to feel it again.

Some symptoms of over-exercising include:

- *Decrease in performance*
- *Loss of coordination*
- *An increased chance of becoming winded after a short amount of time*
- *Having trouble completing a workout*
- *Headaches*
- *Loss of appetite*
- *Constant achy muscles*
- *More susceptibility to illness*
- *Irritability and depression*
- *Trouble concentrating*
- *Rapid weight loss*
- *Weight gain*
- *A raised resting heart rate (especially in the morning)*

It is important to know the signs to keep over-exercising from becoming an issue. Below is a sample chart that will show you what a weekly exercise schedule can look like. You can create your own schedule using the blank chart provided at the end of this chapter.

Monday	Tuesday	Wednesday	Thursday	Friday
Light Warm-up (8-10 minutes)	Cardio Warm-up (5-6 minutes)	REST	Cardio Warm-up (5-6 minutes)	Light Warm-up (8-10 minutes)
Light Stretching (5-8 minutes)	Low Intensity Cardio (10-15 minutes)		Low Intensity Cardio (10-15 minutes)	Light Stretching (5-8 minutes)
Intense Exercise (20-30 minutes)	Intense Stretching (10-15 minutes)		Intense Stretching (10-15 minutes)	Intense Exercise (20-30 minutes)
Intense Stretching (5-10 minutes)	Cool Down (5-10 minutes)		Cool Down (5-10 minutes)	Intense Stretching (5-10 minutes)
Cool Down (4-5 minutes)				Cool Down (4-5 minutes)

Warming up increases your body's internal temperature and allows the synovial fluid to start moving in the joints. By warming up your body's internal temperature, you are helping prevent tears and pulls in your muscles. You want to get your heart pumping before you start to exercise. To warm up, use similar, gentler movements that you will be using in your workout.

Stretching helps release the lactic acid build up in your muscles. It also helps increase the blood flow and aids in flexibility. Make sure you build in light, moderate, and intense stretching into your routine to keep your muscles pliable and healthy.

- *Light stretching* – the stretch is held for only a few seconds; count to 4 then release
- *Moderate stretching* – the stretch is held for 8-10 seconds
- *Intense stretching* – the stretches will be deeper and held for as long as you feel necessary. This type of stretching will help with soreness later. Only perform this type of stretch after your workout is over and your muscles are warm

Cooling down is important for bringing your heart rate back to normal. To cool down, you can perform simple breathing exercises, slow walking, or small, similar movements that you used in your workout. This would also be the time for you to massage out any tight muscles to prevent lactic acid build up and sore muscles.

Make sure you are continuing to stay in shape on vacation or whenever you are not in dance. Putting together a fitness program that incorporates your favorite dance moves as well as other strength training exercises is a great idea for the off season. That way, it will be easier for you to transition back into dance when your break is over.

Now that you know how to exercise properly and what types of exercise to do, we are going to discuss some common injuries that come with being a dancer and how to prevent and treat them.

WEEKLY WORKOUT CHART

MONDAY	TUESDAY	WEDNESDAY	THURSDAY	FRIDAY

Personal Goals and Targets

START DATE: _____ END DATE: _____

MY GOAL

_____
_____
_____
_____
_____
_____

MY PLAN

_____
_____
_____
_____
_____
_____
_____

PHYSICAL ACTIVITY TARGETS

DAILY ACTIVITY	REPETITIONS/TIME

WEEKLY ACTIVITY	REPETITIONS/TIME

EXERCISE TRACKER

DATE			WEEK #	DAY
Time	Type		Intensity	Duration

NOTES FOR TODAY

CHAPTER TWO

Common Dance Injuries

Every dancer and athlete is prone to injuries. It helps to understand the injuries and their symptoms in order for you to properly take care of them the moment they happen. With the knowledge of the symptoms, you can easily diagnose and treat minor injuries with these simple tips. If your injury does not improve within 2-3 days or is painful, swollen, hot, or colored (red or purple), visit your doctor as it may be a more serious injury.

INJURY PREVENTION

The most important thing you need to remember is that maintaining the integrity and health of your connective tissue is key to avoiding injury. *Preventing* injuries is the best way to *avoid* injuries. To keep your connective tissue (ligaments, tendons, etc.) healthy and strong, try drinking a smoothie with Collagen Protein (*store.draxe.com*) after every class or exercise. Collagen is the main structural component in all connective tissue throughout the body. Supplementing with these shakes will help maintain ligament and tendon strength and help you avoid injuries such as tendonitis, strains, and pulls.

Another great way to avoid certain injuries, is by making sure you are getting enough of the essential minerals that your body needs to function. When you are low on minerals such as magnesium, calcium, manganese, and iron, your muscles, connective tissue, nerves, and blood have a hard time functioning properly which can cause injuries like tears, sprains, and fractures.

The best ways, other than eating the minerals in your food sources, is by walking on the beach, adding sea salt to foods, and soaking your feet in warm, Himalayan sea salt baths. Sea salt contains all essential minerals due to the fact that it is not processed as heavily as table salt.

IGNORING THE PAIN

Pain is your body's way of telling you that something is not right. When you feel pain, stop whatever you are doing immediately, especially when the pain is coming from joints. Dull, achy pain is usually pain coming from sore muscles and is not necessarily bad, whereas sharp, shooting pain can mean something is seriously injured. Find where the pain is coming from and treat it properly. Make sure you are stretching and cooling down appropriately to avoid injuries and over-exercising.

Even though there are ways of preventing injuries, sometimes they are unavoidable. In the next few sections we will discuss how you can treat various minor injuries. Please remember that if you have a severe injury, you must visit a doctor as they may result in future complications if left untreated.

TIGHT MUSCLES, PULLS, STRAINS, AND SPASMS

Neck Strain or Spasm

A strain is a small tear in the muscle fibers from overstretching or overuse, while a spasm is a contraction of the muscle in order to prevent further injury to the area.

When you have a spasm, the muscles tighten to the point of immobility. To protect the injured muscles, a spasm might occur. If you use your neck in spite of a spasm, it could turn into a strain.

If a dancer does not properly protect the spine when arching the head and neck, the muscles in the neck can get tight and easily strained during choreography. Michael Kelly Bruce, associate professor at The Ohio State University suggests that you *"'lengthen the neck rather than collapse it…using the image of…a long, graceful arch.'"*

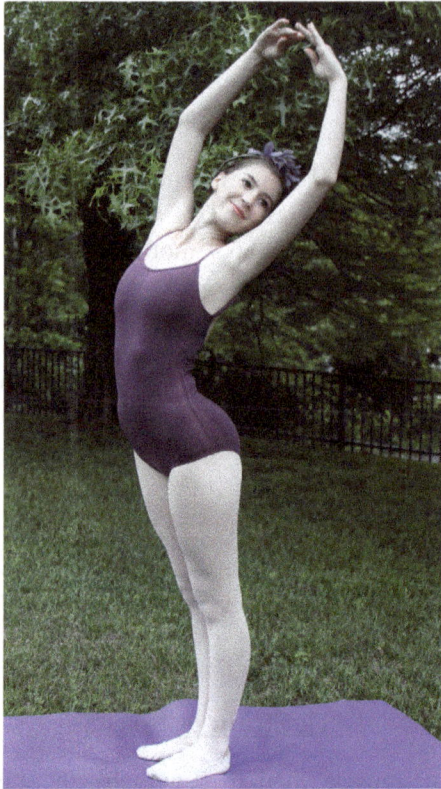

If your neck becomes painful when you move it, you should visit a doctor as you might have a severe neck strain. Severe neck strains are caused by a complete tear in the muscle.

To avoid overly tight muscles that could eventually turn into a strain, massage your neck regularly after class to remove tension. You can also roll your neck from side to side stretching out the muscles.

Start with your head leaning to the right, slowly bring your chin down to your chest, and then to the left. You never want to circle it to the back because it puts too much pressure on the vertebra.

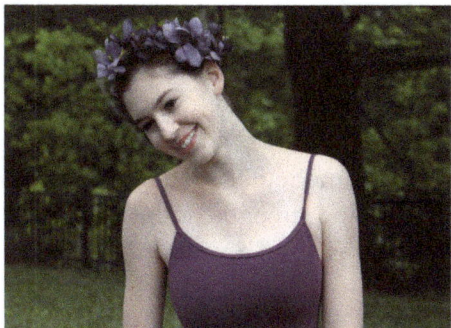

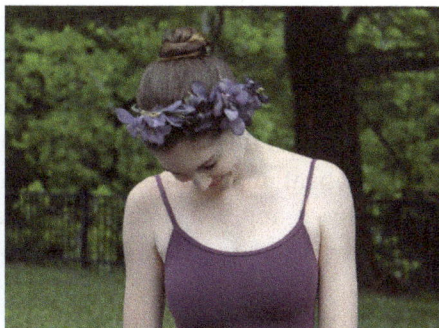

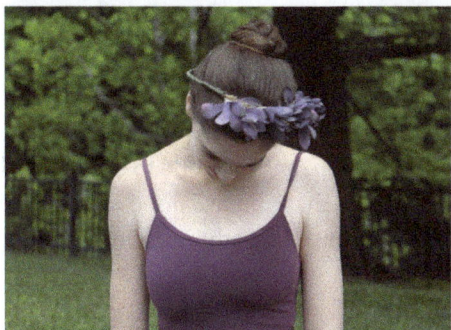

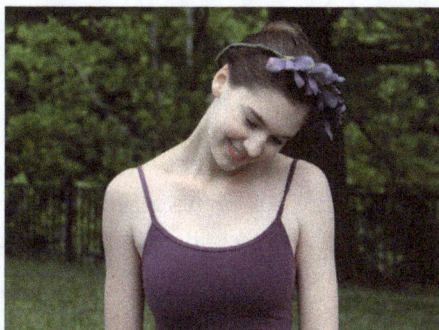

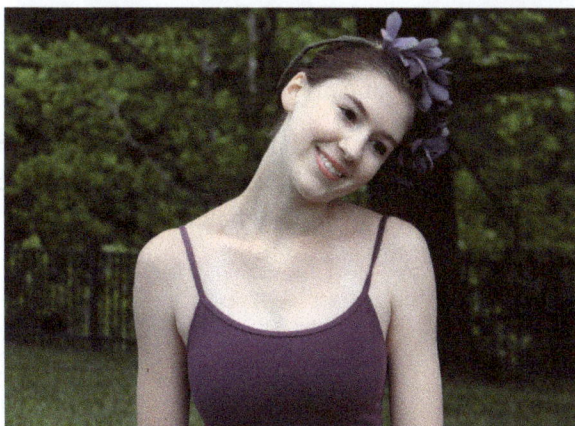

Rest your neck until mobility comes back and it is no longer painful. It also helps to alternate ice and heat. Place an ice pack on the affected area for 15 minutes and then switch to heat for 15 minutes. Protect your skin by placing a towel under the ice and heat packs.

To promote faster healing, an MIT or TDP lamp can be placed over the tight and painful areas. An MIT (mineral infrared therapy) lamp or a TDP lamp creates mineral infrared waves that can treat minor ailments including back pain, shoulder pain, joint pain, and arthritis. It helps to improve circulation, metabolism, and strengthens the immune system. This type of lamp is commonly used by therapists and acupuncturists.

Back Strain or Spasm

Just like a neck strain, a back strain is due to overstretching and minor tearing of the muscle fibers. As with any strain, if the pain is unbearable, visit your doctor.

If you do not have enough core strength, your back will be more prone to strains and spasms. Make sure you are using proper technique and that you are not over-stretching or over-arching your back. Back spasms are usually caused by tight muscles and by jumping with poor alignment.

The best way to prevent back strains and spasms is to make sure that your back is flexible. Try doing some light back flexibility exercises to gain a wider range of movement. Make sure you have a strong core as this will take some of the pressure off your lower back, and do static stretching after each exercise routine or class.

One stretch you can do to increase back flexibility, is a back bend against the wall. Walk slowly down a wall until you reach the bottom and hold it there for a couple of seconds, then walk back up. Do not try this if you already have a back strain.

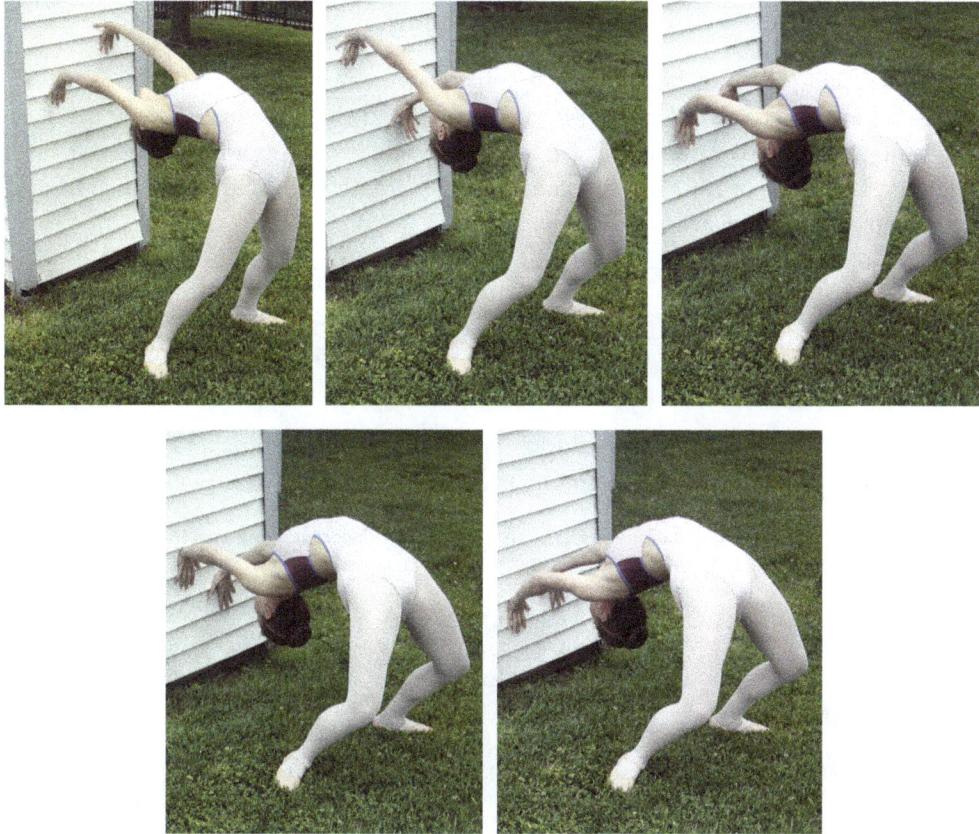

I also recommend massaging your back after every class. It will help you by releasing any tension you have built up during class and it will also help with the healing process. The easiest way to massage your own back is by using a tennis ball.

> Lay on the floor with the ball under your tight muscles and gently roll up and down, back and forth. If it is too painful or tight, use a foam roller instead. If you have a really tight muscle, leave the ball or roller in that area for a few seconds to help the muscle fibers release. Do not hold it too long because bruising may occur, and remember to relax as you roll out the muscle.

Rest is very important for any injury, especially if you find yourself to be slightly stiff. When you have full range back, you can return to regular exercising and dancing.

Snapping Hip Syndrome

Sometimes called "dancer's hip", snapping hip syndrome occurs when the IT band becomes inflamed. The muscles around the outside of the hip weaken and you can feel the IT band snapping over the upper leg bone. You will hear a popping sound when you swing your leg, walk, or run. The constant rubbing over the bone can cause the IT band to become inflamed and sore.

For mild cases, R.I.C.E. (rest, ice, compression, and elevation) can be applied as well as natural anti-inflammatories (*discussed at the end of this chapter*). Special stretches can be done to stretch out the muscle and band to relieve some tension and inflammation (see Chapter 3).

Make sure your lower abdominals, adductors, abductors, and hip flexors are strong. Try to avoid turning out with your feet and instead turn out with your hips.

To achieve your natural turnout, stand in parallel. Lift your foot off the ground and turn it out with your hip. Place it on the ground in the turnout and repeat with the other foot.

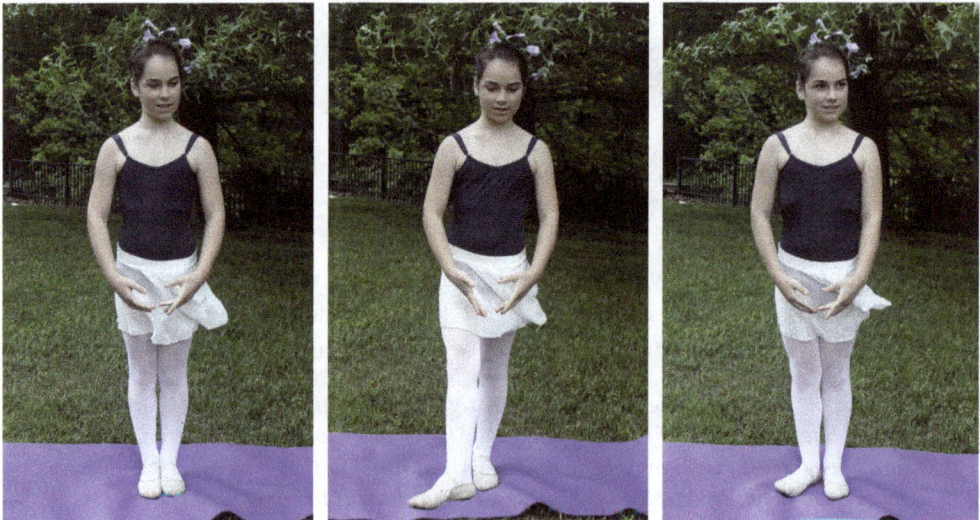

Hamstring Strains

Hamstring strains are usually caused by overstretching. Research has found that someone with a hamstring strain that heals up within 4-6 weeks, is more susceptible to another hamstring strain for 6 months to a year afterward. It is important that you do not overstretch the hamstring when doing exercises such as an Arabesque penchée.

R.I.C.E. can be applied to the hamstring if painful. Exercises that can help with the healing process include swimming, walking in the water, stationary bicycle, and light stretching.

When stretching, start with a bent leg before stretching with a straight leg. This will help with hamstring mobility and will lower your chance for injury.

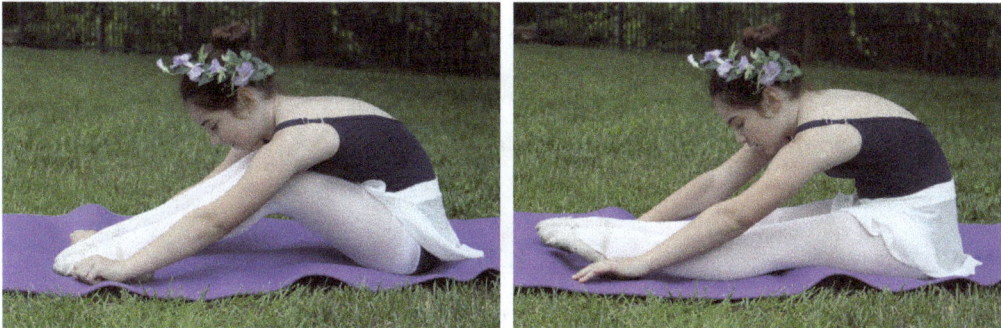

Tight Iliotibial (IT) Band

The iliotibial band is located on the outside of your thigh. Sometimes too much flexion or inadequate warm-up can cause the IT band to become tight and painful. If you are sickling while walking, running, or dancing, it can put stress on the IT band. Knee pain that radiates up to the hip, weakness, or instability in the quadriceps are good indicators that you have a tight IT band.

You can use a foam roller to gently release tension and to keep the IT band loose and stretched. If it is too painful to use a roller, remove some of your body weight by supporting yourself with the opposite leg and your arms.

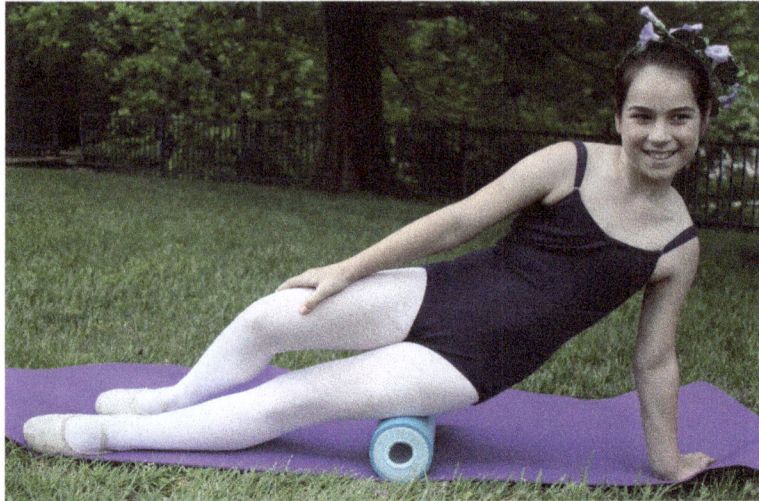

Rest and apply ice for about 20 minutes 2-3x a day.

ACL Tear

The ACL provides stability for the knee and prevents the leg from bending the other way. It is located under the patella (*knee cap*). Tearing of the ACL can occur due to landing from a jump with a stiff leg or twisting the knee outward. You will hear a popping, your knee will swell up immediately, and it will be unstable. Discontinue any activity on that leg in order to prevent cartilage damage. Visit your doctor immediately if this happens as you might need to have surgery.

If you have stability in your knee while performing regular activities and the cartilage is undamaged, surgery may not be required. However, you might need to wear a knee brace and go through some physical therapy to aid in range of motion.

Because tendons and ligaments do not heal very fast on their own, it is very important that you get this kind of injury checked out by a doctor immediately. To help strengthen your tendons and connective tissue, *Standard Process* offers a supplement that aids in their rebuilding and repair functions. The supplement is called *Ligaplex I* and can be found online at *standardprocess.com*.

Patellofemoral Pain Syndrome

When the quadriceps are weak and you have tight hamstrings and calf muscles, it can cause pressure under the knees. The pressure can cause the protective cartilage on the patella to lose its shock absorbing ability. You will feel pain when bending your knees and sometimes you will even experience weakness in the knees.

The best way to prevent this from happening would be to massage your muscles after class to make sure they are not tight. Try to avoid sitting, squatting, or kneeling for long periods of time and stay away from exercises that require bending of the knees. Knee braces, ice, rest, and physical therapy are also helpful ways to allow your knees to heal.

Meniscus Knee Tear

The meniscus cushions and stabilizes the knee joint. If there is too much twisting of the knees during a movement, improper landing during a jump, or forced turnout, the cartilage in the knee can tear. Rolling out your knees, amenorrhea, and restricted caloric intake are also causes.

Symptoms include pain, swelling, difficulty bending and straightening, and a tendency to lock up. The best way to treat this would be to apply rest, ice, compression, and elevation. Visit a doctor if the pain gets worse or it lasts more than 3-5 days. If locking occurs, it means that the cartilage was damaged and might need surgery.

Water Under the Knee

When the fluid in the joint (*synovial fluid*) is over-produced, it causes swelling within the joint itself. The knee will be painful to stand or walk on for long periods of time. This is an overuse injury and can get worse if not properly rested as there is a possibility that it could turn into Bursitis.

Bursitis is when the bursa, a tiny fluid-filled sac that reduces the friction between joints, gets inflamed. This often happens because of overuse or a previous injury. Some of the symptoms include pain, swelling around the joint, warmth, tenderness, and pain with joint motion.

If the swelling and pain persist and gets worse fast, there may be infection and you should see a doctor. If there is bruising around the area, you will need to visit a doctor as there might be damaged capillaries that could result in infection.

Ice for 15-20 minutes 4-5 times a day. Wrap lightly with an ACE bandage or use a knee brace and elevate it above your heart. Natural anti-inflammatories can be used to reduce the inflammation. To help quicken the healing process, you can put your knee under the M.I.T. machine that we discussed earlier, for 40-60 minutes.

If you are prone to water under the knee, try to avoid squats, lunges, and any other strenuous knee bending exercises. Take a break from any knee movement for about a week or two.

Lateral Ankle Sprain

A lateral ankle sprain is a tear that occurs in a ligament when landing unbalanced out of a jump. It is caused by poor technique, fatigue, weak ankles, weak lower leg muscles, and rolling in of the ankles. Symptoms include swelling, soreness, stiffness, and bruising around the area.

The best ways to treat it would be the R.I.C.E. treatment 3x a day for 10-20 minutes and light resistance training. An ankle wrap is also a great way to relieve some of the pressure.

A compress of chamomile essential oil can be placed over inflamed or sprained joints. Chamomile oil is very calming and contains Azulene, a powerful anti-inflammatory agent.

FRACTURES

Stress fractures are overuse injuries that cause the breakdown of bone forming little breaks or cracks. They are most common in hips, legs, and feet. Depending on the severity of the fracture, it can take up to 8 weeks of recovery time to get back to normal.

When your bones are frequently used, like muscles, they become stronger. However, exercises such as jumping, running, or jogging can cause the bones to become weakened making them more susceptible to fracturing. Amenorrhea, diabetes, osteoporosis, and eating disorders can also cause bone weakness.

You must pay attention to the signs of a stress fracture. Make sure you know what the symptoms are so that you can treat them accordingly.

> _Mild fractures_ are slightly painful with a gradual onset of pain over time. There might be tenderness, heat, and the pain will go away with rest.
>
> _If there is pain that lasts a couple of hours after you have stopped an activity and then subsides, it is a _moderate fracture_. They can usually be taken care of at home with rest for 6-8 weeks along with the R.I.C.E. treatment._
>
> _Severe fractures_ are painful during every day activities and the pain continues while at rest. They should be looked at by a doctor as they may need surgical intervention to help heal.

The best way to prevent stress fractures is by varying your routine. Make sure that you are not putting too much stress on one area of your body when doing strenuous exercises. As I have said before, I strongly recommend that dancers not do a lot of running or jogging as it puts too much pressure on the delicate bones in the feet. As dancers, we need to protect these bones. If you do choose to run, wear good running shoes with enough padding and try to use your thighs more than your lower legs. I also recommend that dancers do interval training and cardio regularly to keep variety in their exercise routine. You do not want to just do ballet all the time.

If you do end up getting a stress fracture, you want to make sure you take the necessary time off to let it heal and to prevent further complications. Dancing on an already compromised bone can lead to a clean break, which means taking more time off to heal than you originally would have if you had just left it alone. Take coconut oil to maintain strong and healthy ligaments and connective tissue (coconut oil is discussed in more detail in the *Health and Nutrition* chapter).

Another great way to help your fracture heal faster is by using *Dr. Christopher's Complete Tissue and Bone*. It penetrates deep to allow the bone to heal properly. Calcium Lactate is a supplement that is also great for building strong and healthy bones. You can find both products on Amazon.

Getting Back to Class

Returning to your normal routine might be exciting but take it slow. You do not want to have future complications so make sure you are not pushing yourself too hard. Try swimming to build up strength in your muscles and bones. It is an easy and gentle way to get back into action. Make sure you warm up properly before class or any exercise. Do some gentle exercises to get your heart pumping and your body warm without putting stress on the weak bone.

Take natural anti-inflammatories such as Marcozymes. They are much better for your health than over-the-counter drugs. A full list of natural anti-inflammatories is discussed in more detail in the *Natural Anti-Inflammatories* section of this chapter.

One of the best ways to heal quicker is to use an M.I.T (mineral infrared therapy). It is a lamp that you put over the injured area. It provides relief to muscular aches and pains caused by arthritis and soft tissue injuries, alleviates inflammation and edema from soft tissue injuries, assists in the healing of skin disorders, balances the nervous system, promotes the healing effects on internal organs, and treats bone fractures. This device is great for any type of injury whether it is a muscle pull or a mild fracture.

TENDONITIS

Tendons connect muscles to bone and are made up of collagen fibers and water. They are wrapped in synovial sheaths with synovial fluid to reduce friction and to provide blood supply. Inadequate time for recovery can cause an overuse injury called tendonitis. If the tendon is constantly overloaded and never rested or taken care of, the fibers can start to break down resulting in a tear.

> *Mild tendonitis is when you feel pain during an exercise but the pain goes away immediately after stopping. There may also be slight inflammation and swelling.*
>
> *Moderate tendonitis is when the pain continues for a couple of hours after the activity has been finished and then goes away. Inflammation increases and it becomes slightly more painful for you to dance or perform.*
>
> *Severe tendonitis is when the pain continues throughout the day and night. The pain may also be present during everyday activities instead of just during dance. Inflammation increases significantly and can even be tender and red. This is when you should consult your doctor.*

There are several types of tendonitis that occur in different areas of the body. I will only discuss the three most common among dancers and most athletes.

Rotator Cuff Tendonitis

Also called pitcher's shoulder or swimmer's shoulder, this type of tendonitis is an overuse injury that occurs in the shoulder joint. If you are using your arms too much during choreography, it can create little tears in the upper-arm tendons and muscles.

If you develop this type of tendonitis, there will be pain between the scapula and the rotator cuff when the arms are lifted. There will also be some swelling, stiffness, clicking sound during movement, and loss of mobility and strength.

Make sure you are maintaining good posture and avoid carrying heavy items with one arm. The best treatment other than natural anti-inflammatories would be the R.I.C.E. method and limited movement (sling). Stretching and increasing flexibility will help your shoulder get back to normal faster (see Chapter 3). Physical therapy is also an option for severe cases.

Achilles Tendonitis

Achilles tendonitis is caused by overuse through excessive training in a short period of time. Dancing on a tight calf muscle can also cause the Achilles tendon to tire. It is also caused by poor technique, high instep, hard flooring, shallow plies, weak thighs, and landing on the balls of the feet instead of the whole foot when jumping. When performing plies in class, make sure they are deep enough to stretch the Achilles, giving it somewhat of a break.

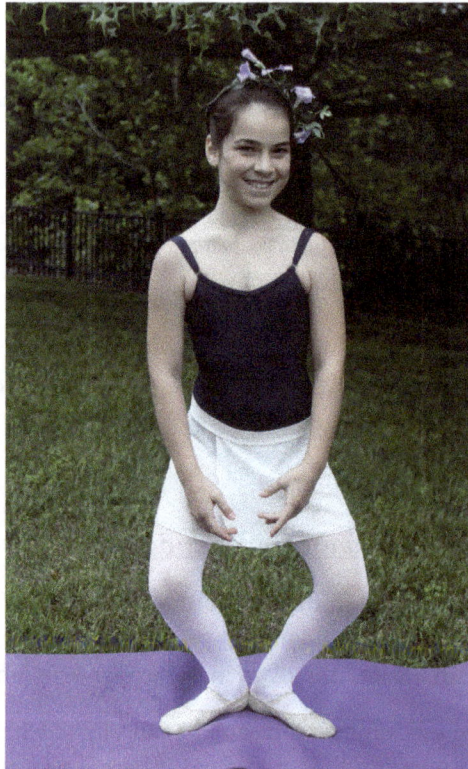

Treatment includes R.I.C.E. and strengthening the arches, calves, and quads. To reduce any swelling, elevate your foot above your heart. If it is a severe case, physical therapy and immobilization may be required.

Posterior Tibial Tendonitis

The posterior tibial muscle is located on the inside of the ankle and connects to the back of the shin bone. The tibial tendon attaches this muscle to the bones of the foot, is located on the back of the leg, and turns in toward the inner ankle attaching to the bone adjacent the arch.

The tibial tendon tires out when the arch falls in turnout. This can cause shin splints and excessive ankle rolling. Some causes include over-exercise (running, dancing, swimming, etc.) and insufficient warm-up and stretching.

There can be pain on the inner side of the foot and ankle and can often feel like an ankle sprain. There will be swelling and pain along the course of the posterior tendon, weakness when turning the toes inward, and inability to stand on toes. If left untreated, the arch can fall and become flat and the toes will start to turn outward.

When exercising, keep your stride balanced and aligned and strengthen your arches (see Chapter 10). Posterior tibial tendonitis is most common with people who have previously sprained their ankle.

Anti-inflammatories and R.I.C.E. are the best ways to aid in the healing process. Sometimes casts are required to properly heal. If the tendonitis is bad enough, an MRI and surgery may be required.

Tendonitis can reoccur if not properly rested and taken care of. Make sure you remain immobile for 2-4 weeks depending on the severity. To reduce the reoccurrence, warm up properly before class and gently stretch after class holding each stretch for at least 20 seconds. Stop if you feel pain as it could lead to a worse condition.

THE DANGERS OF USING NSAIDS

NSAIDs or non-steroidal anti-inflammatory drugs, can be detrimental to a person's health and wellbeing for many reasons. They quickly reduce the pain and inflammation making them one of the most important items in a dancer's bag. However, even though it may seem as if the pain is gone, NSAIDs only mask the pain by blocking the production of a chemical called, prostaglandins.

When you take an Advil, Aleve, or Aspirin, the prostaglandin levels are hindered. Because the formation of this chemical is hindered, the body's inflammatory process is less likely to shut down properly. To heal, we need the prostaglandins to repair the injured tissue and to form collagen fibers for the muscles.

Taking too many NSAIDs can cause a heightened risk of ulcers, gastrointestinal bleeding, kidney disease, heart attack, and stroke. They delay the healing processes creating a more serious injury in the future. If taken too often, they can cause serious damage to the liver and in more serious cases, the brain. Believe it or not, even rubbing the gel on your toes affects you because your skin absorbs everything. It is okay to take an ibuprofen every now and then, but try to limit yourself to only taking them if absolutely necessary.

NATURAL ANTI-INFLAMMATORIES

Because of the high risk involved in taking over-the-counter anti-inflammatories, it is best to look for healthier alternatives. Some of these choices can be put in your foods, some can be made into a tea, and others can be taken as a daily supplement.

Supplements

Please remember to consult your doctor before taking any supplements on your own.

Neprinol AFD—

Neprinol AFD is a dietary supplement that contains serrapeptase, nattokinase, protease, lipase, bromelain, papain, rutin, alma, coenzyme Q10 (CoQ10), and magnesium. "*This unique blend of all-natural enzyme and antioxidants is formulated to support healthy levels of fibrin as well as other EBPs* (endogenous blood particles). *The formula works systemically, or throughout the body to support healthy heart and immune function.*"

Fibrin is a protein formed in the human body that comprises things such as scar tissue and blood clots. Fibrin plays a vital role in the healing process, however, if there is an overproduction of fibrin, it can lead to dangerous and potentially life-threatening blood clots.

The enzyme plasmin is the body's natural way of removing excess amounts of fibrin. It acts as a natural blood thinner and helps to maintain the body's normal blood solvency by removing excess accumulated proteins. Neprinol AFD assists in removing these excess amounts of proteins and helps break down extra fibrin that has built up in the blood.

Marcozymes —

These enzymes contain proteolytic enzymes, which are a special kind of enzyme that helps break long chains of proteins into smaller amino acids. This break down of inflammation promotes healing and rapidly decreases swelling.

The main ingredients in Marcozymes include pancreatin – a combination of digestive enzymes that aid in digestion of fats, proteins, and sugars. Papain – a natural ingredient found in papaya that helps treat inflammation and fluid retention. Lastly, bromelain – proteolytic enzymes found in pineapples which help treat inflammation and pain.

Serretia —

This supplement contains serrapepatase which has been proven to decrease recovery times from injuries and can reduce swelling up to 5 times faster than using ice. It can also promote normal breathing, post-surgical recovery, and a healthy response to injury.

Serretia digests any dead tissue that can accumulate due to an injury, thus, swelling and pain is reduced enhancing the ability to heal. This supplement is great when taken alongside Neprinol AFD.

Wobenzym N —

Wobenzym N is a blend of pancreatin, papain, bromelain, trypsin, and chymotrypsin that work together to provide temporary relief from aches, pain, and muscle soreness. It also supports overall joint and tendon health and helps to increase flexibility and mobility within those areas. The blend of enzymes break down proteins that cause inflammation within the body.

Spices and Herbs

Cumin —

Usually used to flavor many Middle Eastern dishes, cumin is much more than just a spice. It contains minerals such as calcium, magnesium, iron, zinc, and some B vitamins that can aid in anti-bacterial, anti-septic, anti-viral, anti-oxidant, anti-parasitic, digestive, and anti-inflammatory responses. This spice was originally used in traditional Ayervedic medicine in India to treat dyspepsia (indigestion) and diarrhea.

Not only does cumin aid in digestion, it is also great for clearing the lymphatic system of excess toxins, relieving nausea, colic, bloating, headaches, migraines, bronchial spasms, coughing, asthma, increases circulation, is a thyroid stimulant, and boosts energy levels and appetite. Another wonderful attribute is the fact that cumin can help relieve muscle pain from strains or pulls.

Black cumin is different than regular cumin and has different uses. The oil from the seed can help cure hemorrhoids, fever, and stomach upset. Black cumin contains bronchodilatory, hypotensive, anti-bacterial, analgesic (pain relieving), anti-inflammatory, and immunopotentiating properties.

Cumin has also been proven to aid in cancer prevention and treatment. Tumors in the stomach, colon, and cervix have been effectively decreased from taking cumin. The cumin helps stop the buildup of carcinogens and eliminates cancer-causing substances.

For bronchial issues, dilute some cumin powder or cumin oil and apply a poultice to the chest. Nausea can be treated by brewing some cumin tea and sipping at it until the nausea has passed. Cumin essential oil can be diffused to help control bacterial diseases such as Helicobacter pylori (H. pylori). It can also be added to your foods for a delicious flavor boost.

Thyme —

Thyme is one of my absolute favorite herbs! It has such a mild and earthy taste that is wonderful in most recipes. Containing anti-bacterial, anti-inflammatory, anti-histamine, and anti-anaphylactic properties, this herb is a power house. Thymol, which is the active ingredient in thyme, is also a fungicide and increases the omega 3 fats in the brain, kidneys, and heart.

Thyme offers health benefits for people with rheumatoid arthritis, asthma, and inflammatory acne. This is because thymol blocks TBK1 which is linked to most inflammatory diseases. It also has been proven to cause cell death within cancer cells and helps fight H. pylori.

A tincture of thyme and myrrh can fight against bacterium that causes cystic acne, and is proven to be more effective than benzoyl peroxide, the active ingredient in most acne creams.

Sage —

Sage can be used dry or fresh in foods as well as in oil form. It has been discovered that sage extracts have the potential to enhance memory in Alzheimer patients. Sage contains anti-inflammatory, anti-septic, and anti-microbial properties that can help with gastrointestinal issues and diabetes.

Tea made from brewed sage leaves can help treat dysmenorrhea, diarrhea, gastritis, tonsillitis, and sore throat.

Turmeric —

A great anti-inflammatory spice, turmeric, is most common in curry. Turmeric contains curcumin which has powerful antioxidant with anti-inflammatory properties. Curcumin can inhibit the molecules that cause inflammation. It neutralizes free radicals and increases the body's anti-oxidant activity.

Alzheimer's and depression are caused by low levels of a growth hormone, BDNF. Curcumin can reverse the effects by increasing the levels of this hormone. It can also boost the neurotransmitters dopamine and serotonin (happy hormone) in the brain.

Finally, curcumin also improves the function of the lining of the blood vessels, preventing heart disease. It also regulates blood pressure and prevents clotting. Curcumin can also help with anti-aging which is pretty cool.

You can either add turmeric to your food or you can take curcumin as a supplement, for extra strength.

Ginger —

Well known for its ability to relieve nausea and improve digestion, ginger root is packed with phenolic compounds, vitamins, and minerals to help your body repair itself and improve digestion. Ginger is also great for increasing immunity and can even reduce muscle pain caused by inflammation.

The main compound in ginger is called gingerol. Gingerol helps fight infections including yeast infections, gum inflammation, and gingivitis. It stops bacteria growth and contains curcumin which is excellent for immunity. Ginger can also lower blood cholesterol and reduce menstrual cramps and indigestion.

Add dried/powdered ginger to recipes, add sliced ginger to teas, or just snack on some sugared ginger slices to gain the extra immune support you need for the day.

Rosemary—

Rosemary contains an anti-oxidant called rosmarinic acid as well as many health benefitting oils such as cineol, camphene, borneol, bornyl, acetate, a-pinene, and more. All of these oils are rich in anti-inflammatory, anti-allergic, anti-fungal, and anti-septic properties. Not only does rosemary have many healthy oils in it, this herb is also rich in folic acid, pantothenic acid, pyridoxine, vitamin A, iron, potassium, calcium, vitamin C, manganese, copper, magnesium, and riboflavin.

Rosemary oil is used to soothe gout, rheumatism, and neuralgic conditions. A tea made of brewed rosemary leaves can remedy headaches, colds, and depression.

Foods

Kelp—

Brown algae extract is the best type of kelp as it is a complex carbohydrate. It contains flucoidan which has anti-inflammatory, anti-tumor, and anti-oxidative properties. Studies have shown that brown algae can help with liver and lung cancer as well as promote slow fat absorption, helps you to stay full longer, and maintains weight loss.

Make sure you only get organic in order to avoid pesticides and other chemicals. Other types of kelp to try are Kombu, wakame, and arame.

Wild-Caught Salmon—

Salmon is rich in omega-3 fatty acids, two of them being EPA (eicosapentaenoic acid) and DHA (docosahexaenoic acid). These fatty acids help to prevent heart disease and some cancers, as well as reduce the symptoms of certain autoimmune diseases and psychological disorders. Salmon is best when eaten two times a week.

Not a fan of salmon? Sardines, mackerel, anchovies, freshly ground flaxseeds, and walnuts all contain ALA (alpha-linolenic acid) which eventually convert to EPA and DHA, essentially providing the same health benefits.

Avoid purchasing fish that has been canned in polyunsaturated oils such as safflower, vegetable, soybean, corn, and sunflower. These types of oils are linked to inflammatory responses causing heart disease and cancer, and will counteract the health benefits of the fish.

Shitake Mushrooms –

These mushrooms contain high amounts of copper accompanied by amino and fatty acids. Our bodies are not able to synthesize copper so it is important that we get a regular supply of it through our diets. Copper can help maintain a healthy heart and prevent heart disease when it is in constant supply.

Shitake mushrooms also contain pantothenic acid, selenium, riboflavin, niacin, zinc, and manganese. Vitamins B2, B5, and B6 work to break down inflammation, tumors, bad bacteria, viruses, and fungus. Other great mushrooms to consider are maitake, enoki, and oyster as they are all cancer fighting and immune boosting.

Green Tea –

Green tea contains polyphenols which are powerful anti-oxidants that reduce the formation of free radicals, protecting the cells and molecules from damage. Flavonoids, potent and natural anti-inflammatories that reduce the risk of heart disease and cancer, can also be found in green tea.

It also contains the amino acid L-theanine which decreases anxiety and increases the hormone, dopamine, in the brain. Because of the high amounts of anti-oxidants, green tea boosts the metabolic rate making it easier for you to lose weight, kills bacteria that can lead to tooth decay and cavities, lowers your risk of infection, lowers your risk of type II diabetes, cardiovascular disease, heart disease, and Alzheimer's.

Papaya –

Contains papain which is a protein-digesting enzyme as well as vitamins C and E. They reduce inflammation, improve digestion, and heal burns. Pineapple is also a great choice for improving digestion and aiding in trauma, healing, and swelling. Avoid dried fruits that contain sulfur dioxide as they are linked to respiratory disease.

Blueberry –

Rich in anti-oxidants like Anthocyanin, vitamin C, B complex, vitamin E, vitamin A, copper, selenium, zinc, and iron, blueberries are great for boosting the immune system and fighting infections. These little berries have also been proven to aid in brain health, heart health, digestion, and can even improve vision. Blueberries also contain phytonutrients and antioxidants that help with cancer and dementia. Blackberries, cranberries, strawberries, and raspberries also contain these anti-oxidants.

Extra Virgin Olive Oil—

Oleocanthal, and phytonutrient found in olive oil, reduces inflammation. Polyphenols protect the heart and blood vessels. Monounsaturated fats that help with asthma and rheumatoid arthritis can also be found in olive oil as well as, vitamin E which is great for immunity and healthy skin. Avocados are also a great choice for eating healthy fats.

Purchase your oil in its purest form and avoid all partially hydrogenated oils.

Broccoli—

Broccoli is extremely good for you! It is high in potassium which is great for brain function, muscular growth, and regulated blood pressure. Broccoli is anti-inflammatory, anti-cancer with phytonutrients such as sulforaphane which helps the body get rid of potentially carcinogenic compounds. Cauliflower is also a good choice for aiding in the body's detoxification.

Sweet Potato—

A complex carbohydrate, sweet potato contains betacarotene, manganese, vitamin B6 and C, and dietary fiber all of which are great for strong immunity, aiding in digestion, bone and tooth formation, and aiding in blood cell formation. Sweet potatoes also contain vitamins A, B2, B6, C, E, and K, calcium, folate, iron, magnesium, manganese, potassium, and tryptophan. Spinach is also great for anti-inflammatory and anti-oxidative flavonoids and carotenoids.

SPEEDY HEALING

Our bodies have a natural healing process but sometimes it needs a little help to maintain a constant state of homeostasis. Eating well, drinking lots of water, and taking (or eating) natural anti-inflammatories can help with this natural process. Most active people are prone to some sort of injury. The best way to help those injuries heal faster is by taking care of them at the first sign.

Remember to consult your doctor if your injury persists or gets worse within a couple of days. I also recommend doing your own research on everything that I have discussed in this chapter. It is important to be informed about these and other injuries in order to know how to properly diagnose and take care of yourself.

CHAPTER THREE

Stretching Techniques for Flexibility and Strength

Flexibility and strength go hand-in-hand when it comes to maintaining healthy

muscles and joints. It is important to balance both flexibility and strength to avoid injuries like dislocated joints and strained muscles. If you are overly flexible you need to focus on strengthening the muscles to avoid over stretching. Balancing both and being able to control your flexibility is important for being physically fit.

SECRETS TO FLEXIBILITY

Did you know that your flexibility does not only come from stretching and

lengthening your muscles? A lot of people do not fully understand where their flexibility comes from and how to properly maintain it. Your joints control all the major movements that happen throughout your body so it is important that they are flexible and strong. It will not matter how flexible and long your muscles are if your joints and fascia are tight.

Increasing the range of motion (*ROM*) in your joints will help with flexibility gains. You can do this by performing stretches and exercises that use the full ROM of a given joint.

Neck:

Sitting tall, stretch your neck to the right, bringing your ear to your shoulder. Hold that stretch for 4 counts, then slowly bring your neck to your chest and hold for another 4 counts. Roll your neck to the left, bringing your left ear to your shoulder and hold for 4 counts. Repeat this stretch 4 times.

Sitting tall in the same position, rotate your head to look to the right and hold for 4 counts. Turn your head to face the left, holding for 4 counts. Repeat this movement 4 times.

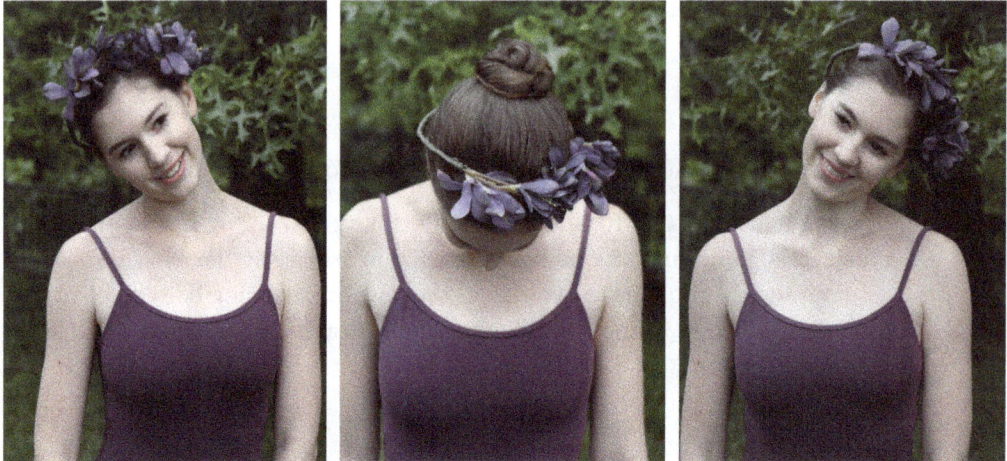

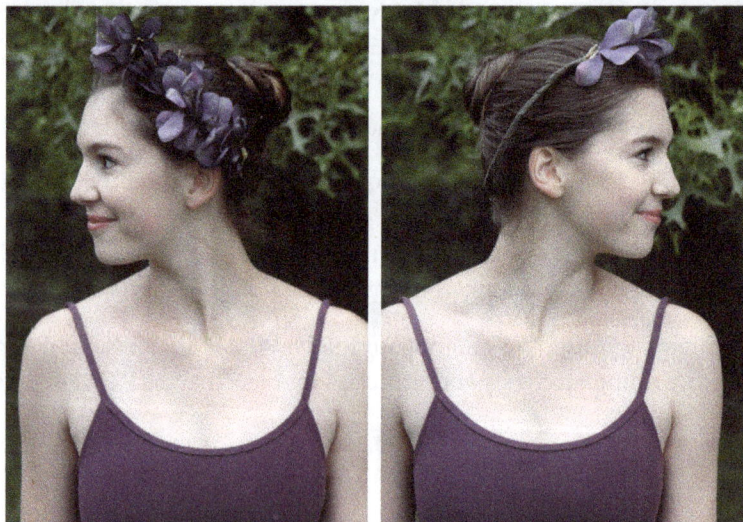

Shoulders:

Stand next to a wall and place your hand on it, keeping your arm in line with your shoulder. Your feet should be just under your hips, with toes facing forward. Gently rotate your shoulder in and out, trying not to move your hand. Repeat this movement 20-40 times and then reverse to the other side.

Sit in a chair, making sure your back is straight. Perform large, slow circles with your arm, bringing your arm all the way forward, up, back, and down. Repeat this movement 4 times and then reverse it. Start the circles on the other arm.

Sitting tall, start rolling your shoulders in a shrugging motion. Roll them up to your ears, back, down, and forward. Perform this movement 4 times then reverse the circles.

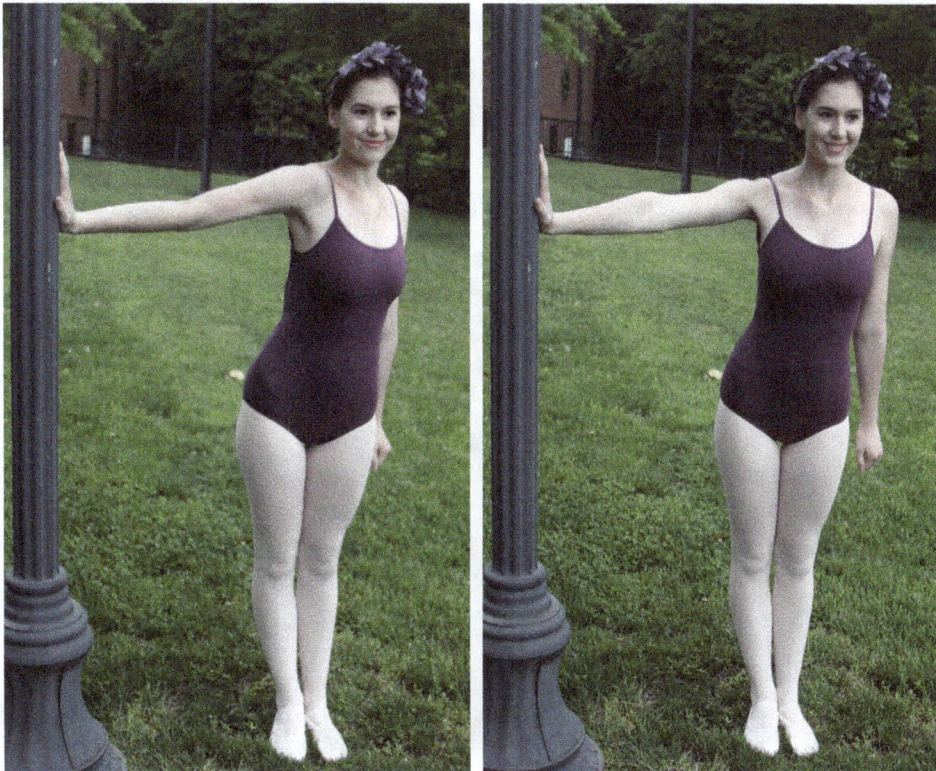

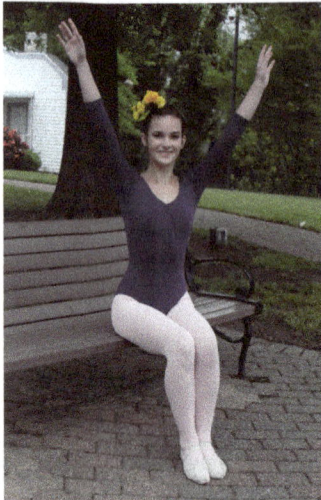 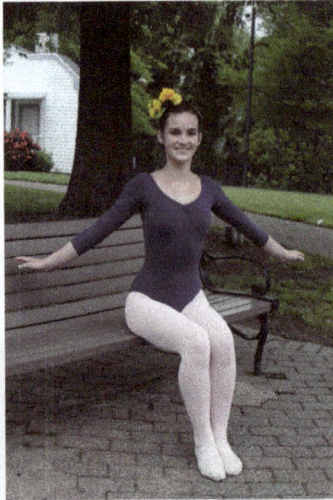 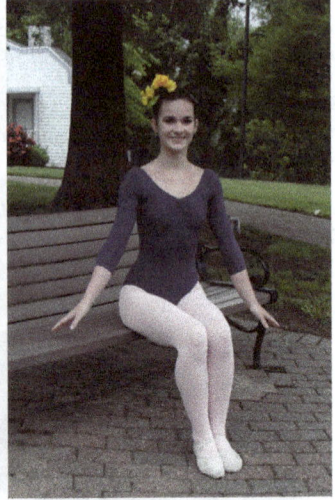

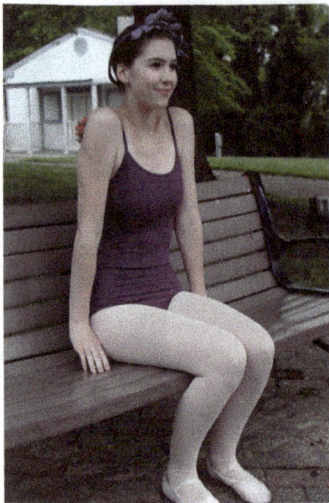 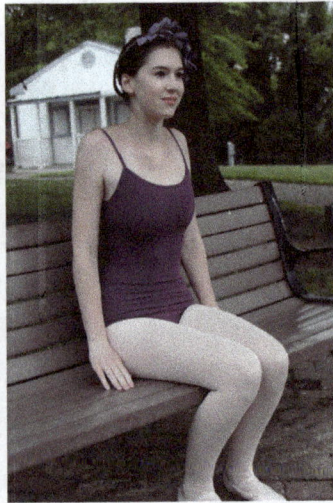 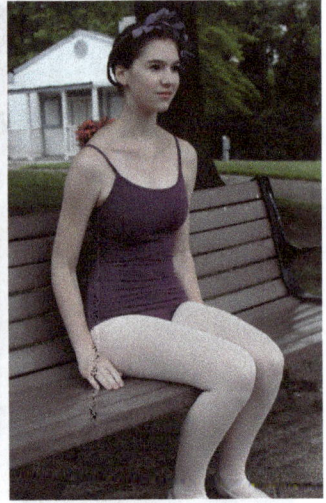

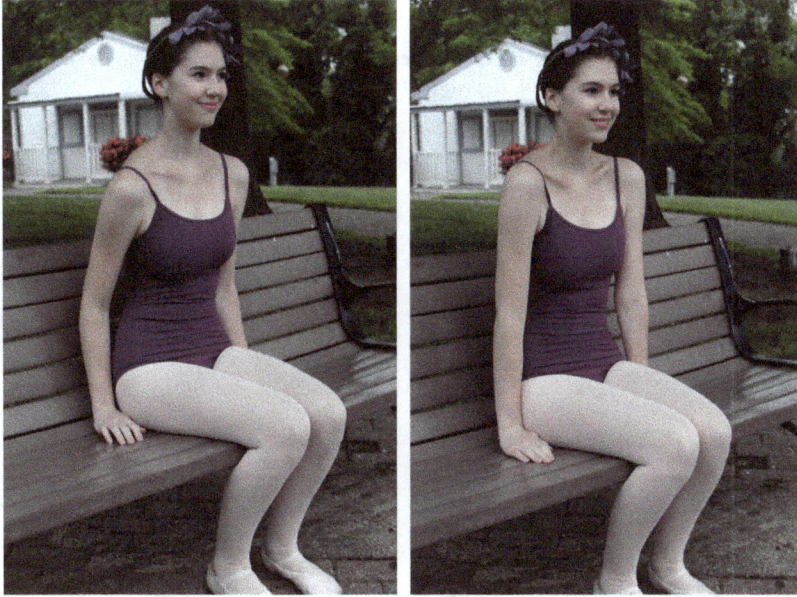

Hips:

Stand holding onto the wall or a chair. Lift your right leg to hip height, keeping it bent and in front of your body. Open your leg, still bent, to the side as far as you can. Lower your toe to the floor, straightening your leg, then raise your leg up and bent to the side. Bring it to the front again and lower straightened. Repeat 3 more times and reverse to the other side.

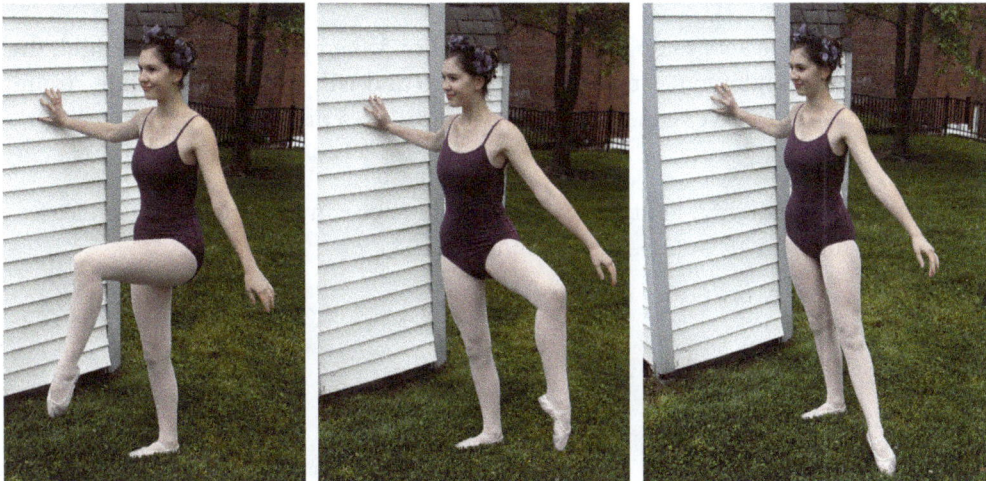

Roll your ankles in slow circles 4 times. To make this exercise more fun, prop one of your ankles on your opposite knee, and draw the alphabet with your foot. Repeat on the other side.

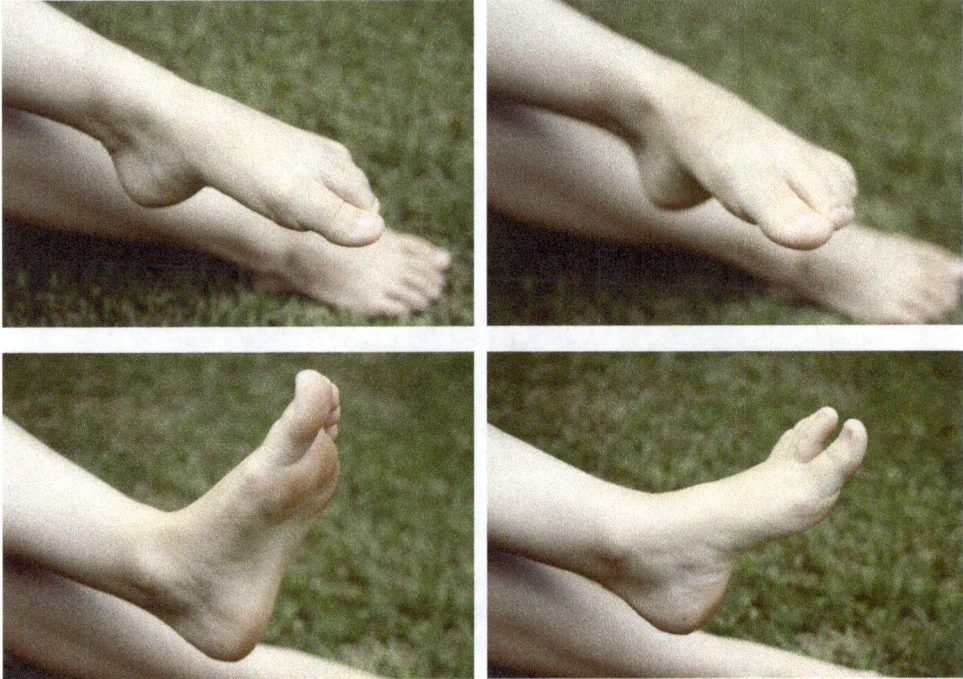

Your nerves also have a lot to do with your flexibility. When your muscles are tight, the nerves running through them can become restricted and will not be able to slide around in their sheaths. Your nerves can also be restricted due to a previous injury or inflammation.

To increase neural mobility, light stretching and massage can help the muscles release tension, allowing the nerves to be able to slide again.

Use a foam roller to gently release tension in various areas of your body. Try rolling your hips, glutes, calves, hamstrings, lats, and shoulders. These points are more vulnerable to tension and are the locations of major nerves that run throughout your body.

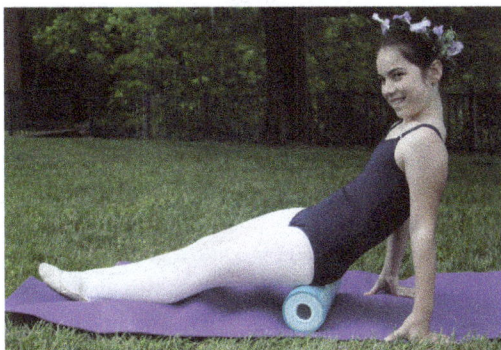

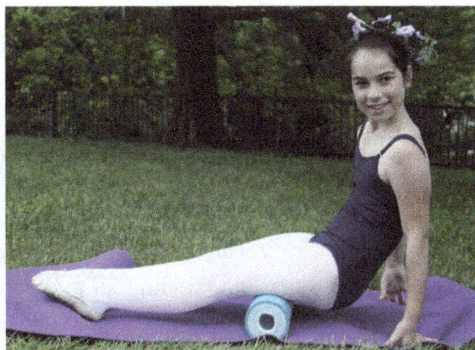

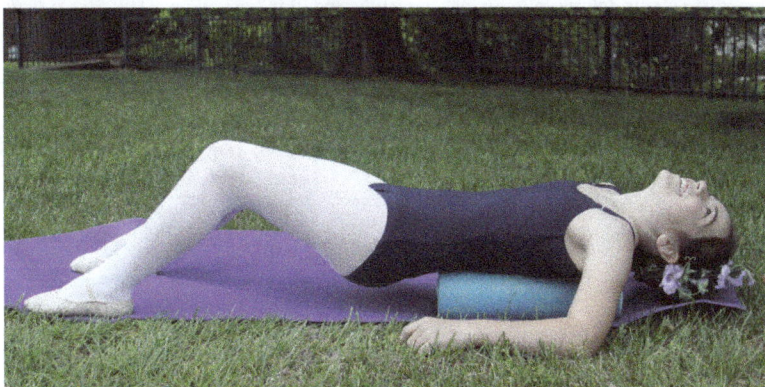

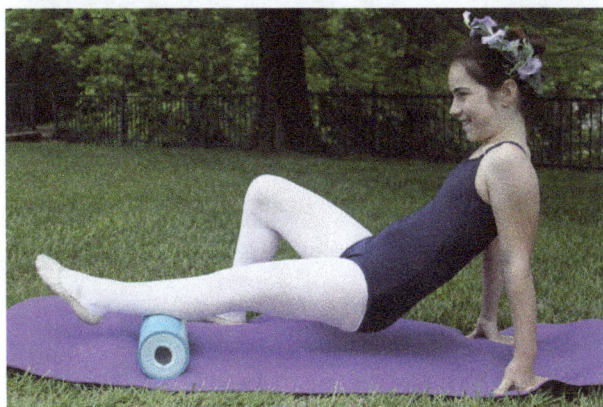

In order to achieve optimal flexibility, you need to release the tension in your muscles and nerves. Stretching both during and after class will help you increase flexibility. You also need to release the fascia surrounding the muscles through massage.

Fascia is a thin layer of tissue that covers your muscles, organs, and nerves. It connects all your body parts together in a web-like network that runs all the way from your head to your toes. Like muscles, fascia can be tight and should be released for optimal flexibility. If you are continually stretching and not getting the results you want, then you probably have tight fascia or restricted nerves.

"*It's not that their efforts are incorrect, but there could be something else holding them back,*" says Deborah Vogel, an Oberlin College faculty member, neuromuscular educator, and co-founder of the Center for Dance Medicine in NYC.

Test your flexibility by stretching to your toes, remembering how far you go. Then take a tennis ball and massage the plantar fascia on the bottom of your foot.

Try and touch your toes again, the same way as before. You should have more flexibility in your hamstring, and be able to stretch further.

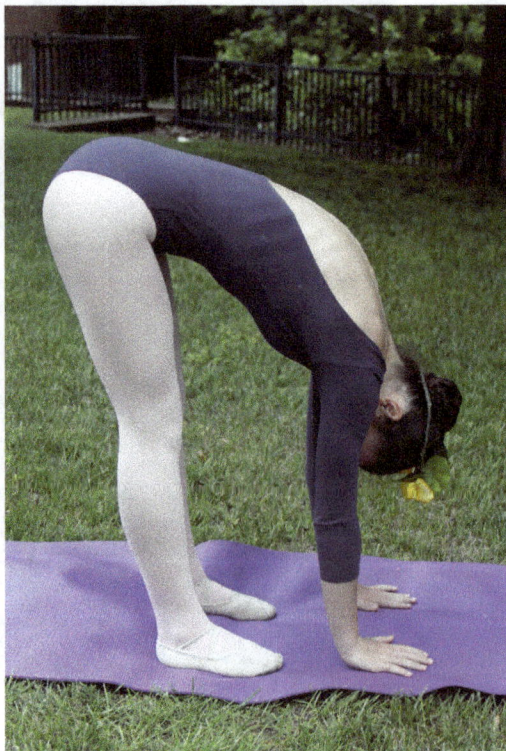

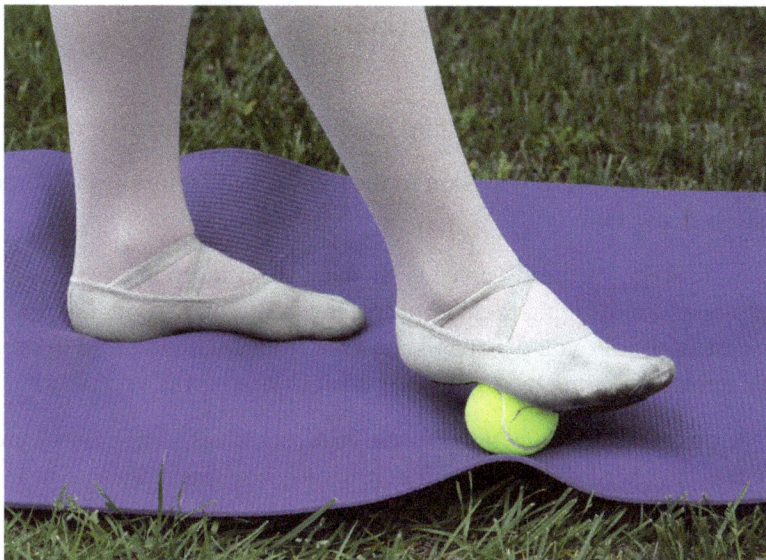

The plantar fascia is connected to fascia that runs up the back of the legs. When you release the tension in your feet, it increases the flexibility all up the back of your legs and hamstrings.

Decreased flexibility in the legs can come from tight shoulders, neck, spine and hips. Releasing this tension can help you stretch further in your legs.

Massage your neck and shoulders to release the tension in your fascia. You can either use a tennis ball or the self-massage techniques provided on the next page.

Drink plenty of water to keep your muscles and nerves healthy. Dehydration can cause your muscles to become brittle and more prone to injury. We will discuss how much water you should drink in the *Health and Nutrition* chapter.

MASSAGE TECHNIQUES

Massage is important to release built up tension in tight, overworked muscles.

Flexibility can be inhibited by any tension in the muscles and joints so it is important to use massage to increase mobility.

Dancing and exercising constantly can cause tension to build up in your muscles if you are not stretching and massaging them appropriately. You want to make sure that you massage your muscles after you dance to keep your muscles pliable and to prevent injury. If your muscles become too tight, it can lead to strains and even tears.

A tennis ball is great for releasing large muscle groups such as your glutes, calves, and back. Do not press too hard as it can result in bruising. Use light pressure in sensitive areas and heavy pressure in areas where the muscles are extra tight and rolled up.

Self-massage for shoulders and neck:

- *Start by first assessing your tension level by rubbing your shoulders, feeling how tight your muscles are. Always remember to adjust the pressure based on how your muscles feel. The massage should never be painful.*
- *If you have a lot of tension on the tops of your shoulders, use your first and gently kneed the muscles with your knuckles. If you do not have much tension, use back and forth motions with your fingers along the muscles.*
- *On the tops of your shoulders, use your fingers to rub the muscles in small circles, moving from the base of the neck to the shoulder.*
- *Massage your shoulders by grabbing the muscles and squeezing and releasing. Gently rub back and forth to release the tension, and to bring blood flow to the muscles.*
- *You can come to the front, near your clavicle, and gently rub small circles from the shoulder to the chest. If you have a lot of tension in one area, you can apply more pressure.*
- *Moving to the back of your shoulders, start pulling the muscles away from the spine with your fingers. Use your fingers to work the muscles surrounding your shoulder blade (scapula).*
- *Moving up your neck, use gentle pressure with the tips of your fingers. Walk your fingers up to your hair line. Press gently at the base of the skull and hold for 4 counts. Release by rubbing your fingers in small circles.*
- *Make sure you are breathing and relaxing as you massage.*

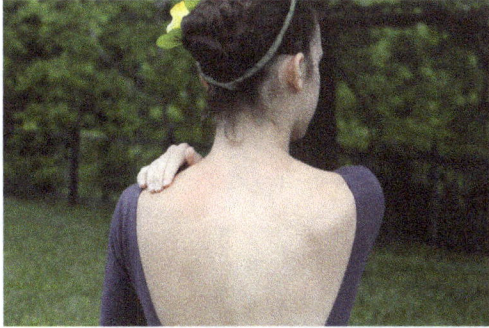
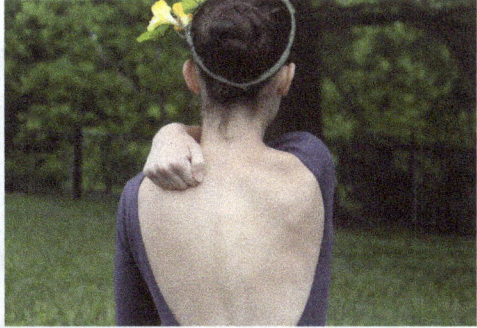
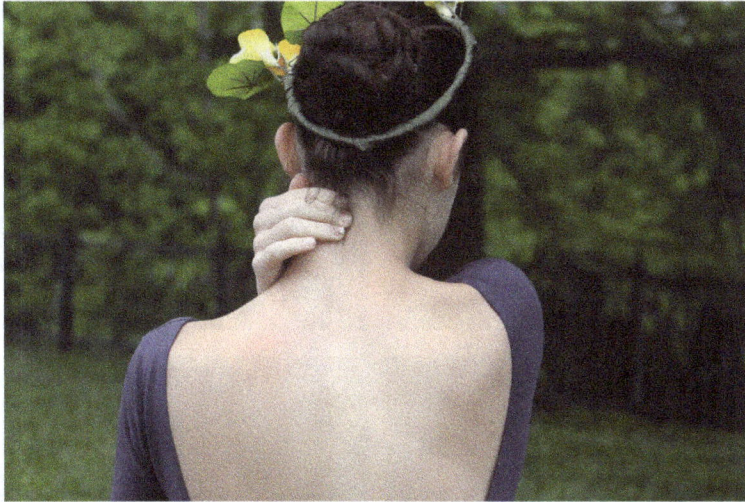
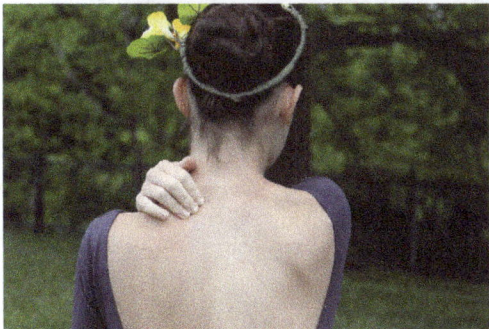
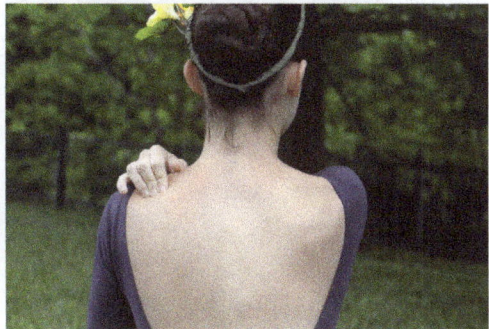

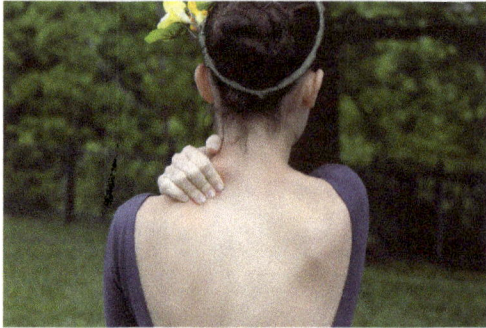 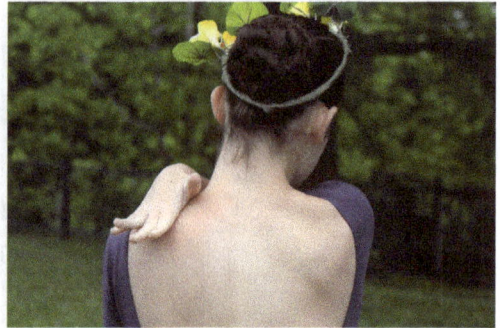

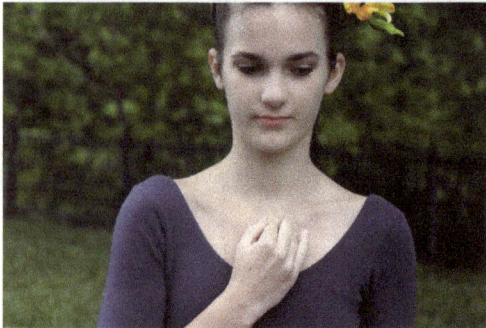 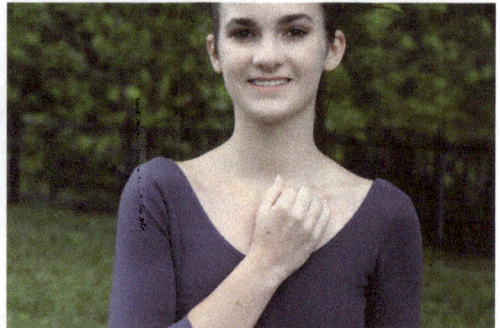

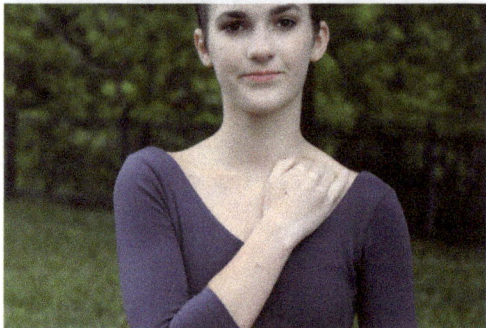 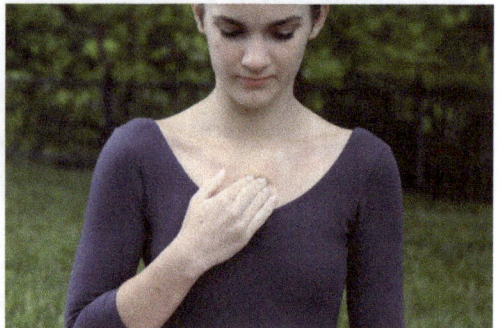

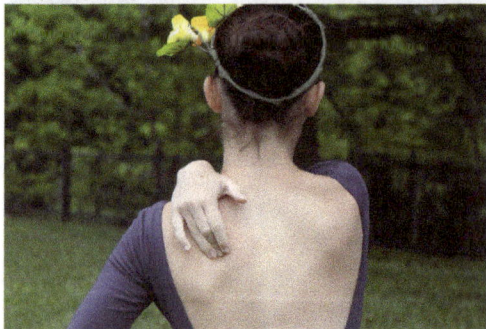 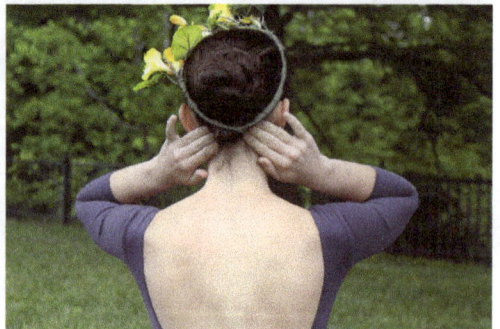

PROPER STRETCHING

Stretching is important for bringing blood and nutrients to the muscles, helping them repair faster. It also removes lactic acid that tends to collect when performing high intensity exercises. Not only does stretching allow the muscles to repair, it also helps gain flexibility and loosens the muscles resulting in less soreness. It is extremely important to know how to stretch properly to avoid any injuries.

Before you perform your stretching routine, make sure you are properly warmed up. If you stretch cold muscles they are more prone to tearing. When you get to class, do not start stretching without a short warm-up. Try jumps such as échappés, changements, or jumping jacks to get your muscles ready to stretch.

Make sure that you are not holding your stretches for too long as it can lengthen and weaken your muscles. When your muscles are lengthened too much, you lose the power in your muscles to perform exercises like grand battements and developpes. Perform static stretches (*holding the stretches for only 4 counts*) before and during exercise.

Do not bounce in your stretches as this can cause tears, making you more vulnerable to injury. If you find that it is difficult to achieve a certain stretch, try stretching with a bent leg first and then straighten it.

Modified stretches:

Modified stretching can be done for especially tight muscles or it you are recovering from a certain injury.

Quadriceps stretch:

Kneel on the floor in a lunge position and gently pull your back foot up toward your back, stretching the front of your back thigh. Release your leg slightly and then gently pull it back in again. Repeat this stretch 4 times on each side, holding the stretch for 8 counts.

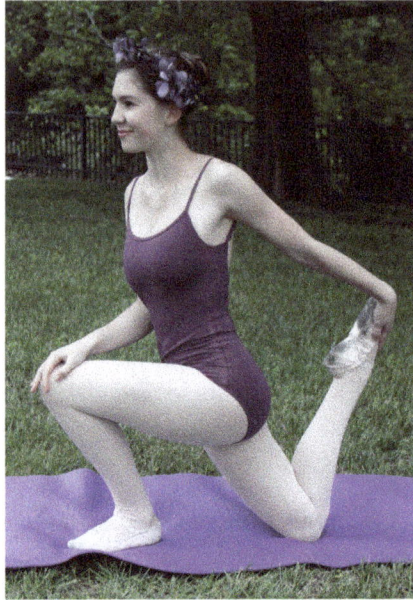

Hip stretch:

Lay on your back with your feet on the floor, knees bent. Bring your right leg up and cross it with the left knee. Gently grab the back of your left leg and pull it in toward your chest, stretching the right hip. Hold this stretch for 10 seconds and then repeat on the other side.

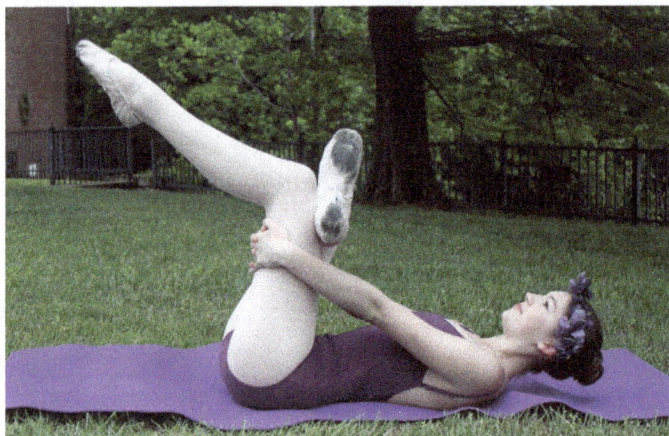

Stretches for fascia mobility:

Releasing the fascia helps improve flexibility, as I have already mentioned previously. These stretches will help release any tension that has built up.

Stretching for tight hips:

Releasing tension in the fascia of the hips will improve your turnout. Sit in a chair with your right leg crossed over your left so that your right ankle crosses over your left thigh. Place your hand on your right leg and gently press the knee down toward the floor.

Make sure your back is straight. Slowly bend forward, still pressing the knee to the floor. Hold this stretch for 10 seconds and release all the way up. For optimal flexibility gains, perform this stretch up to gour times on each side.

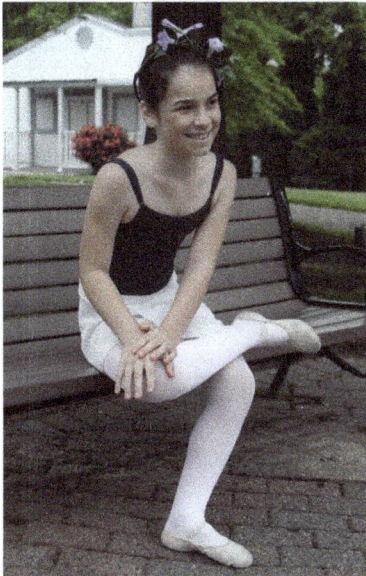

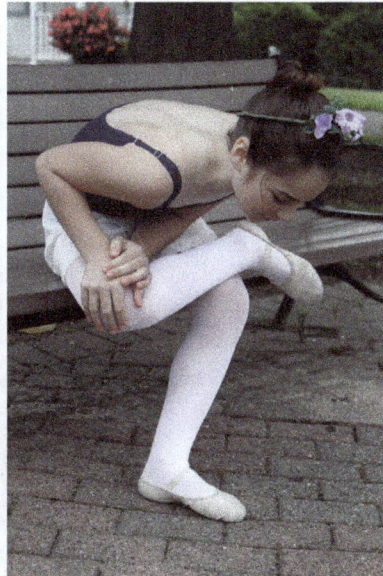

Stand in parallel with your arms raised over your head, and hold your right wrist in your left hand. Squeeze your shoulder blades together, opening the elbows away from each other. Gently bend to the right and rotate so that you are looking to the right. Hold for 10 seconds, then round your lower back to stretch further, and hold that for 10 more seconds. Release and repeat on the other side.

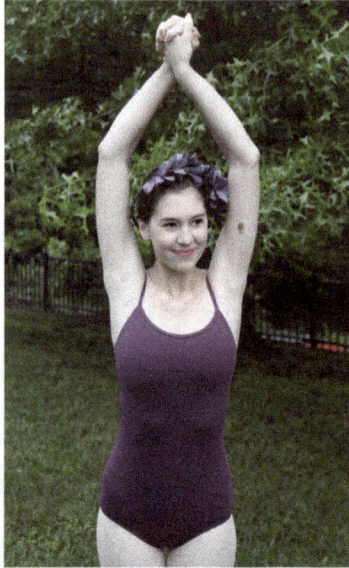

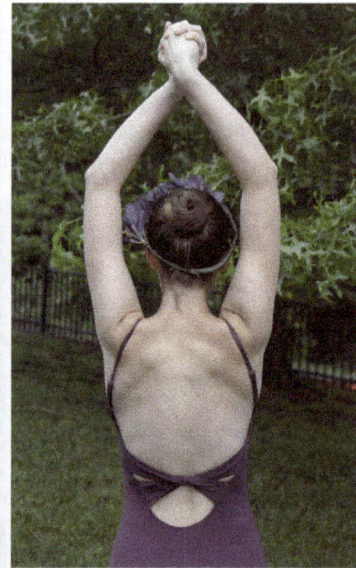

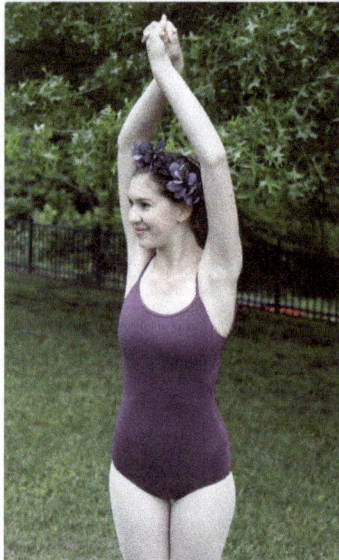

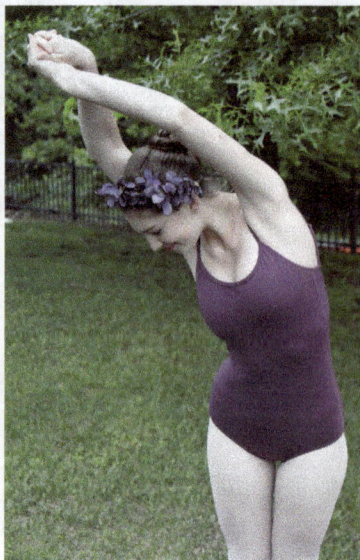

<u>*For hamstring mobility:*</u>

Sit on the floor with right leg straight, and the other bent and relaxed. Roll a towel and wrap it around the arch of your straight leg, keeping your foot flexed. Hold the ends of the towel in each hand, bringing the left arm over your head and resting the right elbow on the floor. Hold the stretch for 10 seconds and repeat on the other side.

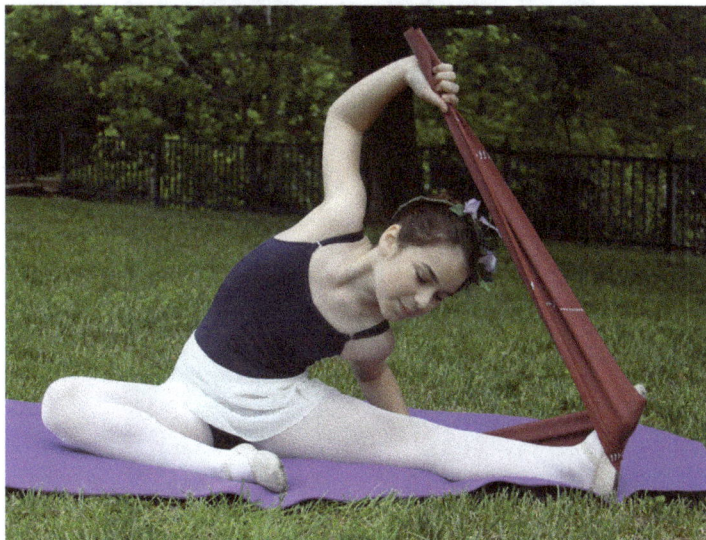

For upper back mobility:

Sit with your legs folded under and your arms overhead. Grab your elbows and bend from the ribcage to the side, and hold for 10 seconds. Release and stretch over again 3 more times. Repeat on the other side.

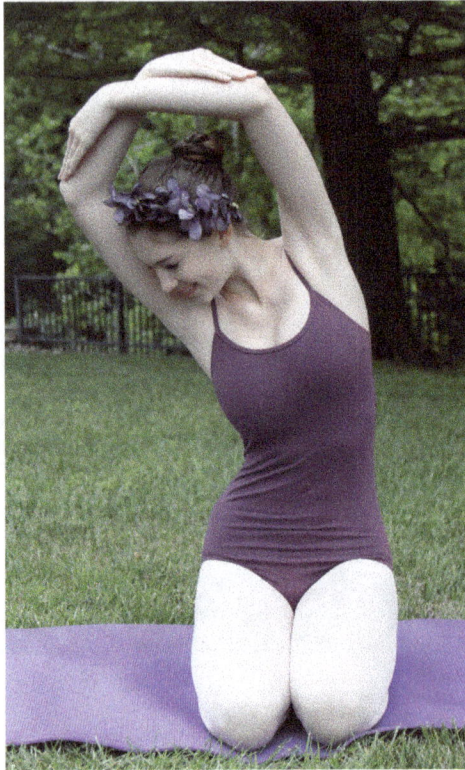

Position yourself on your hands and knees. Arch your back up, bringing your chin to your chest and tucking your tailbone under; hold the stretch for 4 counts. Reverse by arching your spine down, bringing your chin up and lifting your tailbone; hold for 4 more counts. Repeat this stretch 4 times.

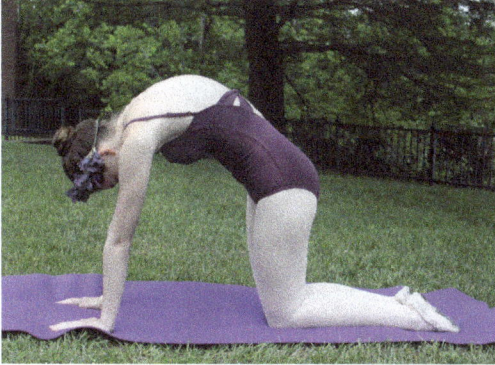

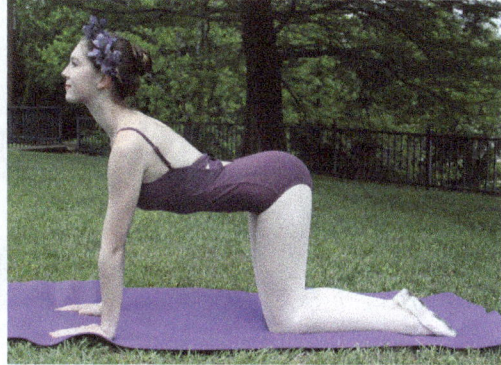

BACK PAIN AND THE BENEFITS OF GOOD POSTURE

Poor posture is the most common cause of back pain along with lack of physical exercise and emotional stress. Back stretches and flexibility mobilizers can align your spine and stretch it out. Making sure you sit with good posture and keeping up with these stretches will help maintain back flexibility.

Having tight iliopsoas muscles can cause the lower back to curve inward causing an improper alignment of the lumbar vertebrae. The iliopsoas (*psoas*) is a muscle that connects to the lower vertebras of the spine and the top of the femur. Having a job that requires you to sit a lot can cause the psoas to shorten and tighten, promoting bad posture.

Massage can sometimes help release tension that has built up in the psoas, however, since it is such a deep muscle, it can be difficult to get at. The best way to release tension in that muscle is to stretch it gently 2-3 times a week until you feel relief.

Lay face down on the edge of your bed, keeping one foot on the floor and the other stretched out on the bed. Prop yourself up on your elbows and start bringing the foot that is on the edge up to your head, as far as possible. Loop a towel or TheraBand around the foot that is on the bed. Gently pull the strap, bringing your foot toward your back and hold the stretch for 30 seconds.

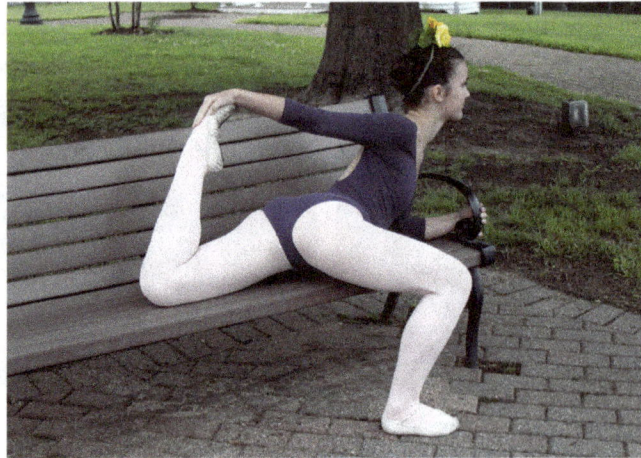

Another muscle that can cause lower back pain is the quadratus lumborum. The quadratus lumborum (QL) connects to the last rib and the top of the hip bone. When it is tight, the QL can cause radiating pain and poor alignment of the lumbar vertebrae.

To stretch out the QL, start by laying on your back with your arms stretched out at your sides. Bend your right leg to your chest, placing your left hand on your knee. Gently lower your knee to the left as far as it will go, keeping your shoulders on the floor. To increase the stretch, turn your head the opposite direction of the stretch. Hold for 30 seconds and gently return to facing upright. Repeat on the other side.

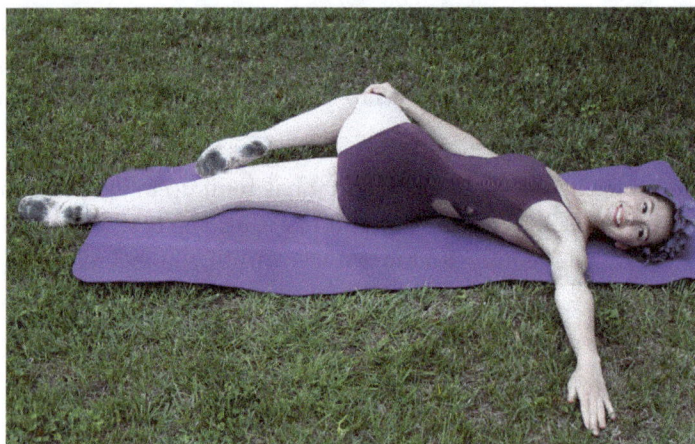

When you are maintaining proper posture, you keep the bones of your spine and hips properly aligned, decreasing the possibility of lower back pain. It also aids in normal joint movement, muscular flexibility, and balance between both sides of your body.

PART TWO

Healthy Dancer

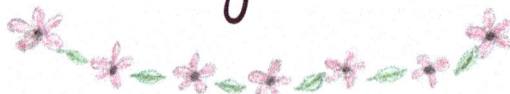

CHAPTER FOUR

Effective Weight Control

For dancers, especially young dancers, weight can often times be a constant reminder of their imperfections within the dance world. Historically, ballerinas were categorized as having long, slender arms and legs, a small head, long neck, and a short torso. This type of body shape was thought to create long and expressive lines on the stage during performances.

Unfortunately, this vision of the "perfect" ballerina has caused many mental and physical health issues in the lives of many dancers. These young girls are thrown into a highly competitive and demanding environment that is constantly assessing their physical appearance and weight. All of this is made worse by the mental and physical demands of dance training on a daily basis.

Dancers with already low self-esteem are more likely to fall into an eating disorder or depression because of their weight or body type. Not only are they competing with fellow dancers, they are also competing with themselves and their own physical appearance. The worst thing that these young girls can do is compare themselves with others.

"Comparison is the thief of joy." –Theodore Roosevelt

Not every person is built the same. Even though most young, aspiring ballerinas strive to achieve the prima ballerina image, not all of them will get to the point where they fit into this "perfect" mold. Young dancers need to remember that they are still in the process of growing. It is normal for a girl's weight to fluctuate during puberty and this can cause a lot of self-image issues. Having classes available on nutrition and body awareness in addition to their dance training is important for guiding young dancers through these tough times of adolescence.

The great thing about this day and age is that ballet is a constantly changing art form. Quite often we see professional ballerinas pushing the boundaries of dance and physical appearance. Take Misty Copeland for example. She is the first black ballerina to make principle in a renowned company. Misty is also one of just a handful of ballerinas that are built more athletically and not gaunt.

There is always room for improvement in any type of art form or ideal. Dance because it makes you happy. No one has the authority to decide what you should look like to guarantee success. As long as you enjoy it and you believe in yourself, you can achieve anything you set your mind to.

NATURALLY CONTROLLING YOUR WEIGHT

It is important to maintain a healthy weight based on your height and body type,

especially as an athlete. There are simple ways of doing this that will not disrupt your performance. Making small changes to your eating habits and activities will drastically improve your energy levels, weight management, and strength. We will discuss a few here but there will be more thorough suggestions in the *Health and Nutrition* chapter.

Many dancers think that lowering their calorie intake will help them to stay thin. Unfortunately, not eating enough calories can cause fatigue, increased risk of osteoporosis, and will increase healing time. It is vital that athletes are eating enough calories in order to maintain their energy levels and overall health. In fact, most athletes must eat *more* calories than the average person because they are constantly having to refuel their bodies. I find that it is easy to sign up for things like Green Blender (*greenblender.com*) or Daily Harvest (*daily-harvest.com*) which send you the ingredients all ready to add to the blender for a quick smoothie for breakfast or between meals.

Maintaining our bodies must involve providing it with the right fuel. You cannot expect a car to operate without fuel so why must your body be any different? Every vitamin and mineral has a purpose and that is to rebuild and repair. If you do not give your body all the materials it needs it cannot perform properly. Instead it will fail you in the form of disease and injury. Invest in the only body you are given and it will give back in return.

Meals

Eating a high fiber diet can help you stay fuller longer and will clean out your digestive tract. Try and stay away from processed forms of fiber, carbohydrates, and sugar as these will raise your blood sugar levels. Donuts, store-bought breads, canned fruits, and white pasta are examples of processed fiber, carbohydrates, and sugars.

Foods such as cucumbers, raw nuts, carrots, and celery are great choices for a quick snack in between meals. Because you are filling up on these healthy fibers, you will be less likely to need more processed snacks during the day.

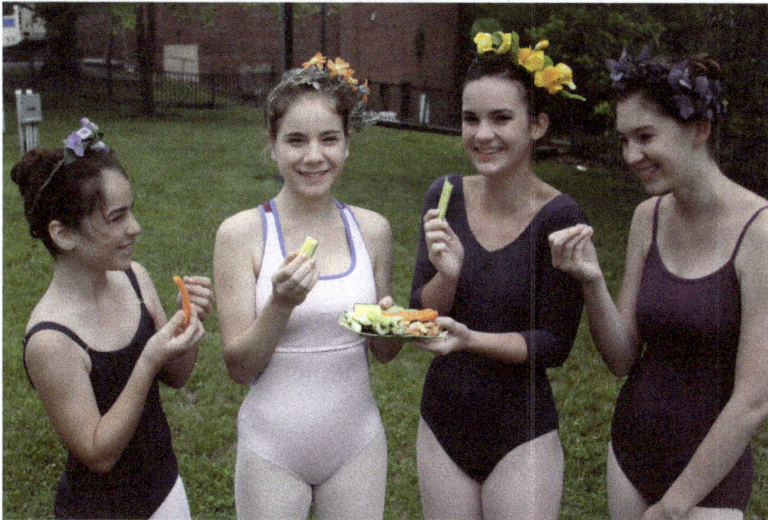

Making a meal plan each week is one of the best ways to prevent unnecessary snacking. If you do need a quick snack, choose something that is healthy and not filled with sugar, excess salt, and carbohydrates. I have shared some of my favorite snack recipes in the next chapter as well as some great tips for packing your snacks and meals to go. Lastly, balance your food groups and mealtimes accordingly to keep you full and to avoid overeating. Ideally you should eat three small meals with small, protein-packed snacks in between.

Try eating organically as much as possible. Organic fruits and vegetables are grown sustainably without the use of pesticides that can cause long-term health issues, allergies, as well as altering hormone levels. Stick to 1-2 fruits a day to keep your insulin levels down and avoid fruit juices. Vegetables and sprouted grains are great for your main source of carbohydrates. Avoid filling up on simple carbohydrates such as bread and crackers.

Watching how many calories you are taking in per day can become an obsession. Food is to be enjoyed and appreciated. Remember it is not your enemy. As you dance, you are burning so many calories that you will need to replenish your body's needs. As long as you are eating healthy and beneficial calories, you will be fine. It is when you start eating foods that are processed and full of sugar and sodium (not including sea salt) that you need to restrict your caloric intake.

Proper amounts of protein and healthy fats will help you stay fuller longer and will eliminate the need for snacking in between meals. It will also help you build muscle much faster. Spices such as cayenne, black pepper, ginseng, mustard, turmeric, ginger, cinnamon, cardamom, and cumin help boost your metabolism making it easier to lose and/or maintain weight. Cinnamon and cumin also help regulate your blood glucose levels, lowering inflammation throughout the body. Black pepper and turmeric help block the formation of fat cells. Ginger relaxes the intestinal tract, and cumin aids in digestion. Teas are excellent ways to get these herbs and spices into your daily routine and it gives you an opportunity to relax.

Choosing one day a week to splurge on a favorite dessert that you can look forward to will make eating healthy for the rest of the week much more bearable. This will help you create goals and will keep your moral up throughout the week.

Another way to remove excess amounts of fat within the body is with coconut oil. Organic, cold-pressed coconut oil has shown to:

- lower and balance hormone levels
- prevent pre-mature aging
- promote healthy skin, nails, and hair
- helps you build muscle
- prevents yeast infections
- protects against Alzheimer's disease
- lowers "bad" cholesterol levels
- maintains the kidneys
- combats inflammation
- boosts the immune system
- lowers and maintains healthy blood sugar levels
- maintains healthy bones and teeth
- and so much more.

Taking one tablespoon of organic coconut oil per day can help you lose any unwanted fat. Although coconut oil is high in fat, the medium chain fatty acids actually help break down the adipose cells in your body. Once those adipose cells are broken down, the fat is then turned into waste that is excreted from the body. Coconut oil can be taken in capsule form, by the spoonful, or added to your foods. Make sure you are buying only the most natural form of coconut oil; organic, non-hydrogenated, extra virgin, and cold-pressed.

Diet and Sugar-Free Drinks and Foods

Avoid sugar and simple carbohydrates as much as possible! They both spike the insulin levels giving you an energy high but a significant crash shortly afterward. When avoiding sugar, a lot of people tend to gravitate toward sugar-free desserts, drinks, and candies. *This is a big no-no.* Diet and sugar-free items are extremely bad for your health. In fact, diet or sugar-free drinks and foods can be worse for your body than actual sugar. Doctors Mehmet Oz and Mike Roizen wrote an article in *The Oregonian* saying,

"[E]ven with FDA approval, conflicting and often bothersome research about calorie-free sweeteners keeps bubbling to the surface. The latest? Evidence from human studies shows that artificially sweetened drinks are associated with weight gain in adults and teens, and raise risk for diabetes, high blood pressure and heart disease. Some data even suggest that these zero-calorie sips could double the risk for metabolic syndrome, a huge risk factor for diabetes and heart disease. Other recent reports show consumption is linked to higher rates of depression."

The worst artificial sweetener is aspartame. It is constantly being linked to diseases such as certain cancers including leukemia, and Alzheimer's. You can find aspartame in gum, soda, candy, and even ice cream. So, stay away from diet and sugar-free drinks and foods. They are terrible for your health and will *not* help you lose weight.

If you must have something sweet, try sticking to foods that are naturally sweetened. Turbinado sugar, coconut sugar, stevia, honey, maple syrup, and molasses are examples of healthy choices that you can use to sweeten your foods. Even though these are healthier forms of sugar, they still must be eaten in moderation. Your sugar consumption should be limited to about six teaspoons a day, not including fruit.

Weight Watching

Constantly watching the scale is not going to make your weight drop off any faster. It is more discouraging to continually see the same number every time, than to just not weigh yourself at all. Try thinking of staying healthy and strong instead of watching your weight. It is more important to be eating healthy foods, exercising, drinking lots of water, and maintaining a joyful outlook on life.

Staying Calm

Stress is the enemy when it comes to staying healthy. When you are stressed, hormones such as cortisol and adrenaline are released. This causes your heart rate to rise, your blood vessels to dilate, your metabolism decreases, and extra glucose is released into your blood stream to give you more fuel to "fly." This is called "fight or flight." Your body goes into this state of stress when you feel as if you are danger.

We will discuss the effects of too much cortisol in more detail in the *Stress Management* chapter. I have also laid out simple breathing techniques, fun activities, and quotes to help you stay calm and keep your stress levels to a minimum.

MUSCLE WEIGHT & FAT WEIGHT – THE MYTH

It is a common thought amongst avid fitness gurus that muscle weighs more than fat.

However, this is incorrect. If you have a pound of fat and a pound of muscle, will they weigh the same? Of course they will! Because a pound is a pound. Unfortunately, this thought does not make a lot of people feel any better about their weight.

Hopefully this will give you more confidence. Picture a pound of lead and a pound of feathers. The pound of lead will likely be much smaller and take up a lot less space than the pound of feathers. The same can be said about muscle and fat. Muscle takes up a lot less space than fat does making you look much smaller than if you had the same weight in fat.

"I find people make this statement when they put on weight," says Stusek via Kristen Stewart's article on Everyday Health. "One person will say, 'I gained three pounds and I've been working out.' The good-friend response is, 'It's all muscle.' And while this is a very comforting thing to hear, it's just impossible to gain three pounds of muscle in a week. It is common for exercisers to lose fat and gain muscle without a change in body weight, so I understand why people often get frustrated."

There will be times when you will not see a difference on the scale, and that is because you are probably gaining muscle but losing fat. So, you are losing weight, it is just not showing on the scale because you are replacing it with something much better. Having muscle will help boost metabolism making it easier to burn calories faster, will help keep you strong, and your bones dense as you age.

Your focus then needs to be on how you feel and how the muscle appears on your body. When you lose fat, you will start to look thinner because fat takes up more space than muscle does. If you are not seeing a difference on the scale but you are fitting into smaller clothing than you are probably losing fat and gaining muscle. You will also be gaining a more defined shape and curves.

However, muscle is denser than fat. Because of this, there will be certain people who will gain muscle mass and weigh more than they did before they started working out. This does not mean that you are overweight or you have too much fat, it just means that you have a lot of muscle that is weighing you down a little more. You have already lost all the extra fat and now your body is building muscle. This is more likely to happen if you are a weight-lifter or body-builder.

THE RISKS OF BEING UNDERWEIGHT

Being underweight is extremely dangerous and can lead to many health issues, two of which include malnutrition and osteoporosis.

Malnutrition occurs when you fail to supply your body with the necessary nutrients that it needs. Vitamin D deficiency can cause rickets (softening or weakening of the bones), vitamin C deficiency can cause scurvy (swollen, bleeding gums and opening of previously healed wounds), and iron deficiency can cause anemia (lack of healthy red blood cells). These types of deficiencies as well as others can affect how you battle infections, resist and recover from illness, as well as how quickly your wounds heal.

Underweight people tend to have lower bone mass densities than the average person. This can cause osteoporosis, a progressive disease that weakens the bones and makes them more susceptible to breaking and fractures. The reason behind this is usually a lack of vitamin D and calcium. Make sure you are spending enough time in the sun to maintain a healthy amount of vitamin D.

COMMON HEALTH ISSUES FOR DANCERS

As with any athlete, dancers are prone to certain types of health complications. The most common among dancers include lowered immune system, amenorrhea, and nutritional deficiencies.

Lowered Immune System

Low impact exercise daily for up to an hour can increase your immune system, making you less susceptible to infections and certain diseases. However, too much exercise can actually lower your immune system. When you perform intense exercises, cortisol and adrenaline are produced more rapidly. These particular hormones ("stress" hormones) are released in abundance, raising the blood pressure and cholesterol levels, thus suppressing the immune system.

Dancing longer than an hour and a half a day for more than three times a week can wreak havoc on your body. Dancers who are active up to 5 hours a day, 5 days a week are more susceptible to getting sick and are also more susceptible to other types of health issues such as the ones we will talk about next. The best ways to combat over-exercising is to continue fueling your body with healthy proteins to rebuild muscle and by getting plenty of sleep to give your body enough of a break at night. Try to limit your dance training to less than 2 hours a day, 3 days a week for adults and 1 hour a day, 3 days and week for adolescents, if possible.

Amenorrhea

Amenorrhea (uh-men-o-REE-uh) is when a woman has missed consecutive menstrual periods. There are three major contributors to amenorrhea—

- *Excessively low BMI: having a lower-than-normal body mass index (BMI) can disrupt the hormones in your body, making you more susceptible to having amenorrhea. Eating disorders can also contribute to low body weight.*
- *Too much exercise: the constant expenditure of energy during dance can cause a loss in body weight, as well as excessive stress to the body. This can also disrupt hormones, thus potentially stopping or creating an irregular period.*
- *Stress: this one is really important. When you are constantly under a lot of stress, whether physically or mentally, it can alter the function of your hypothalamus—the part of your brain that controls hormones. I offer stress-relieving techniques in the Stress Management chapter.*

The best way to avoid amenorrhea is by taking care of your body. Do not take on too much on a daily basis. Limit the amount of class time you are putting in, to avoid over-exercising. Stay calm and relaxed and do not stress about things.

Nutritional Deficiencies

Nutritional deficiencies are becoming more common within the dance world. This is when your body is not getting enough of the nutrients that it needs to perform properly. There are simple ways to make sure you are getting enough of the necessary nutrients by eating properly and taking multi vitamins.

Most common for dancers is a deficiency in vitamin D. Because dancers spend a lot of time indoors practicing, they are not getting the necessary amount of vitamin D they need from the sun. The best way to get enough vitamin D is by getting 15-20 minutes of sun exposure a couple of times per week between the times of 10 and 2. However, there are times when being in the sun is impossible.

Another way to provide your body with enough vitamin D is by taking a tablespoon of cod liver oil a day. You can also take D3 and K2 supplements, which can be found on *Amazon.com* or in Natural Foods Stores.

"'When you take vitamin D, your body creates more of these vitamin K2-dependent proteins, the proteins that will move the calcium around. They have a lot of potential health benefits. But until the K2 comes in to activate those proteins, those benefits aren't realized. So, really, if you're taking vitamin D, you're creating an increased demand for K2. And vitamin D and K2 work together to strengthen your bones and improve your heart health.'"

Calcium and magnesium deficiencies cause your bones and teeth to weaken and your heart, nerves, and muscles to function incorrectly. This type of deficiency is very dangerous for dancers because they need strong bones to keep their bodies moving and supporting them properly. This does not mean that you should be drinking more milk!

Unless the milk is whole, raw milk, it will not provide as much benefit to you. The best foods to provide you with proper amounts of calcium are whole yogurts such as *Brown Cow*, greens like kale and collards, and sea salt. If you decide to take calcium supplements, it should never be taken on its own because pure calcium can cause heart problems. It must be taken alongside vitamin D and magnesium for it to be beneficial to your body.

To absorb these vitamins properly, you need to add enough healthy fats to your diet. If you are eating foods that are low-fat or fat-free, calcium, magnesium, and vitamin D will do you no good.

Iron deficiency causes anemia which is a blood disorder that causes fatigue and weakness. When your body is low in iron, it is not able to make enough red blood cells making it less efficient to deliver oxygen to your organs and tissues. Maca powder contains iron as well as other important vitamins, and *Dr. Christopher's Cayenne Pepper Extract* (*drchristophersherbs.com*) aids in blood circulation and stimulation.

If you are eating well, getting enough rest, maintaining low stress levels, and staying positive you will be able to find joy in dance. Focus more on the joy of dance rather than your weight. It is more important that you are having fun and eating well than constantly assessing your weight and appearance.

CHAPTER FIVE

Health and Nutrition

Your body needs constant refueling to maintain a healthy body composition. Knowing how and when to eat is just as important as knowing what you should eat to support a healthy lifestyle. Eating properly and staying hydrated is essential to having more energy and endurance, and being less prone to injury.

STAYING HYDRATED

Hydration is one of the most important components to a healthy lifestyle. 75% of Americans suffer from chronic dehydration. Dancers and athletes are especially prone to dehydration because of their constant movement during class.

Your muscles are made up of 75% water, so drinking water helps keep your muscles pliable. When you are dehydrated, your muscles can become brittle and stiff. Proper hydration also helps you maintain a healthy weight by increasing metabolism and by flushing out toxins that can build up in your body.

Every time you drink water, you are aiding your body in joint and tendon lubrication, cell growth, the transport of nutrients throughout the body, digestion, and keeping your intervertebral discs healthy. Your skin will also look moisturized and healthy because water brings oxygen to the cells creating a healthy "glow."

An inactive adult female should be able to drink up to 48-64 oz. (6-8 cups) of water per day. Whereas, an active adult female should be able to drink slightly more in order to replenish the fluid they have lost during exercise.

Berkey water bottles have a filtration system inside so you can take it anywhere with you. This makes it easier when you do not have access to filtered water, especially when you run out of the water you brought with you. (*berkeywater.com*)

A great way to make sure you are drinking enough is by taking a full water bottle with your wherever you go. Marie Scioscia, nutritionist at The Ailey School says *"Dancers who are moving continuously for 60 minutes or more should rehydrate with a half-cup of water every hour."*

Try drinking an 8-oz. cup of water 20-30 minutes before you start your exercise, 8-oz. 30 minutes into your exercise, 8-oz. 60 minutes into your exercise, and another 8-oz. 15-20 minutes after you exercise. Remember not to gulp your water but sip it slowly to avoid stomach upset.

When you start to feel thirsty, it is usually an indicator that you are dehydrated. Drink enough water throughout the day so that you do not feel thirsty. Serious dehydration can result in dizziness, fatigue, cramps, and nausea.

As with not drinking enough water, there are also problems with drinking too much water. Too much water can overload the kidneys as well as cause hyponatremia (HI-po-nay-TREE-mee-a), which is when your body lacks enough healthy sodium. This can cause the cells throughout the body to swell and sometimes burst, which is extremely dangerous to kidney function.

The easiest way to see if you are drinking enough water is to check your urine. It may sound gross, but it will show you what is going on inside your body. If your urine is clear, you are probably drinking too much water. If it is dark amber, you are probably not drinking enough water. The ideal color should be light yellow.

Making Water Interesting

Sometimes water can become a little boring, especially when you are drinking it constantly. There are simple and healthy ways to choose alternatives and to enhance your water's flavor, here are just a few.

Lemon –

Add lemon to your water for a boost of energy. The lemon helps to balance your pH levels, is loaded with potassium, has anticancer properties, aids in digestion, and supports weight loss.

I recommend drinking a glass of lemon water every morning before breakfast. The potassium helps build protein and muscle and by drinking lemon water in the morning, you are aiding in reduced inflammation, better digestion, cleansing your body, clearing your skin, increasing your immune system, and it even gives you a healthy energy boost without the caffeine. You can also drink it warm and add a ¼ teaspoon of cayenne and a teaspoon of honey to it for a great detox drink.

Coconut Water —

Coconut water is the best way to replace electrolytes such as magnesium, calcium, phosphorus, potassium, and sodium after exercise. It is low in sugar and sodium, high in chloride, it helps regulate the body's temperature, boosts the immune system and metabolism, and helps with digestion.

There are many different brands and flavors on the market but I would recommend choosing the purest and most natural product you can find such as *O.N.E.* or *Zico*. Stay away from coconut waters that add sugar or any other sweetener as coconut is sweet on its own.

Coconut water powder can also be found online (*amazon.com*) and contains all the benefits of regular coconut water. Just add a tablespoon to your water and it dissolves. My favorite brand is *ActivZ* as it is both non-GMO and organic.

Mineral Water —

If you like sparkling water, this is a great option for you. I find that when I drink mineral water, my sweet cravings are lessened. Mineral water contains various minerals because it is from a spring. Companies like *Perrier* and *La Croix* offer great flavors but my favorite way to drink sparkling water is by adding fresh squeezed lime juice to the plain *Perrier*. You can find these waters in your local grocery store or online at *perrier.com* and *lacroixwater.com*.

Airborne —

During the cold and flu season, you might need an extra boost to keep your immune system working properly. I recommend taking Airborne after every class. They contain Vitamin C to help support cellular health and immune function, Vitamin E, Vitamin A to promote immunity and provide antioxidants, Zinc to support immune function and provide enzymes and nutrients, and magnesium, also to support immunity.

I have noticed that if I put the effervescent tabs in my water after every class, I get sick less often. My favorite flavor that they offer is the berry flavor, but they also offer citrus, grapefruit, and lemon/lime.

Special Tea—

I love drinking tea especially on cold, wet days or after a long and stressful day at work. There are so many different types of tea that are great for your overall health, but there is just one blend that can be used as a regular supplementation method for normalizing the endocrine system and the production of hormones.

This blend is a mixture of Irish moss, Elder berries, Peppermint, and Iceland moss which can be found on *mountainroseherbs.com.*

Irish moss contains 15 out of 18 of the essential nutrients that your body needs including sodium and potassium iodides which work to help with thyroid function. Elder berries are great for colds, flu, anti-aging, lungs, stomach, and many other things. Peppermint is great for relaxation and calming the digestive system and Iceland moss is rich in antioxidants.

> *You can mix together equal amounts of these four herbs in a jar, and they will keep for about a year. The best way to drink this mixture of herbs is by pouring a heaping tablespoon into a filter or French press and brew as long as you like. It is recommended that you drink 4-5 cups of this tea a day to really see a difference.*

Drinks to Avoid

It is becoming more and more popular to grab a sports drink or vitamin water before, during, and after exercise. The down sides to these types of drinks, however, are many. They are usually very high in sugar and sodium and some even contain deadly artificial sweeteners. Because they are so high in sugar, they can lead to lower levels of energy and weight gain if drunk regularly.

Sugar is a simple carbohydrate; something we will talk about later in this chapter. Because it is a simple carbohydrate, you will experience a sudden burst of energy with a significant crash later on. Most sports drinks also have artificial colors to make them more appealing to consumers. They are basically a soda without the carbonation.

Artificial colors and dyes are extremely bad for your long-term health. Studies have shown that most colorings can cause cancer and allergic reactions. Blue 2 was linked to brain tumors in mice, Green 3 bladder cancer, Yellow 3 can cause allergic reactions, Yellow 6 adrenal gland and kidney cancer, and Red 3 thyroid cancer.

Consider this: one bottle of regular Gatorade has about 200 calories and contains 56 grams of sugar. 200 calories is about the same amount the average person would burn running two miles, and 56 grams of sugar is about the same amount of sugar as two-and-a-half candy bars. That's also nearly three times the amount of sugar the average adult woman is recommended to consume.

So, before you grab a sports drink, think about the long-term consequences and choose water instead. Lemon water, coconut water, or just plain old water are the best choices in the end to stay healthy and hydrated.

THE COMBINED EFFECT OF DIET AND NUTRITION

Diet and nutrition play a huge role in maintaining a healthy lifestyle. Exercise causes the formation of free radicals which are similar to rust on a car. They must be counteracted with antioxidant-rich foods. Eating right will give you more energy, help maintain your endurance levels and proper weight, and even give you a glowing complexion.

Healthy Fats

Fats have received a bad rap for being detrimental to your health, especially if you are trying to lose weight. There is, however, a difference between "good" fats and "bad" fats. "Good" fats come in the forms of fish, avocados, olives, and nuts. These fats are higher in monounsaturated fats and omega-3. "Bad" fats include soy, peanut oil, corn oil, vegetable oil, safflower oil, sunflower oil, and canola oil. The reason why these fats are so bad for you, is because they are usually refined and are high in omega-6 which is highly susceptible to oxidation. This makes them reactive and damaging to the body.

Adding healthy fats to your diet can actually help you lose weight. One of the main reasons why a lot of people cannot seem to lose weight is because they have low thyroid hormone. The thyroid hormone regulates the metabolism. Healthy fats aid in the production of this hormone giving you an extra metabolic boost and in turn, giving you more energy.

Fats high in omega-3s help burn extra body fat while keeping the healthy fats for your body's use and can reduce inflammation. Healthy amounts of cholesterol can also be found in fats and helps with the balancing of hormones.

Finally, fats also help to build muscle, promote brain function, reduce heart disease, and strengthen the immune system. Pasture butter, coconut oil, and olive oil are anti-microbial, anti-fungal, and anti-viral which makes them great for killing off bacteria, pathogens, and preventing infections.

Olive oil —

Olive oil is probably the most popular oil to use in everyday cooking. It is rich in monounsaturated fats and vitamin E which can help reduce the risk of heart disease, aid digestion, lower bad cholesterol levels, aid in brain development, and boost metabolism. Olive oil has anti-inflammatory and anti-microbial properties as well as polyphenols that aid in building strong cell walls and increase the elasticity of arterial walls.

Coconut oil —

Coconut oil contains a plethora of healthy fats that are helpful when dealing with viruses and diseases by creating powerful anti-microbial and anti-fungal agents. Its anti-oxidant properties help with skin issues such as eczema and psoriasis. Coconut oil contains vitamins E and K as well as iron which work together to rebuild proteins in the hair making is shiny and soft and can help with regrowth. Rubbed on the scalp, coconut oil removes dandruff and keeps your scalp healthy.

Lauric acid in the coconut oil helps lower cholesterol levels and high blood pressure. Coconut oil also helps the endocrine system function, increases the metabolic rate making it easier to lose weight, aids in digestion, helps control blood insulin levels, and improves the body's ability to absorb certain minerals.

Lastly, coconut oil is anti-fungal, anti-bacterial, and anti-viral giving you an extra immune boost, and prevents tooth decay and plaque formation.

Flaxseed oil—

Flaxseeds are high in fiber making digestion easier, but the oil also has other amazing benefits. It boosts the immune system, decreases cholesterol levels for a healthy heart, reduces inflammation, regulates hormones, and lowers blood pressure.

Flaxseed oil is high in omega-3s that work to prevent plaque buildup in the arteries. Sterols in the oil prevent free radical buildup and can even improve eye health. Flax also aids in hormone balancing due to the lignans found in the oil.

Flaxseeds can also be ground and added to baked goods or on top of oatmeal. Grind only as much as you will need and then refrigerate the rest to prevent them from going rancid.

Sesame oil—

Sesame seed oil has anti-bacterial properties to help eliminate pathogens, is rich in zinc and magnesium, contains tyrosine which is connected to the secretion of serotonin in the brain helping to boost your mood, has fatty acids such as sesamol and sesamin which help with cardiovascular health, and contains copper and calcium for healthy bone growth.

It eliminates hair loss, can be used as a sunscreen to protect the skin from dangerous toxins, whitens teeth, reduces plaque buildup, aids in the production of red blood cells, and helps with circulation and metabolism.

Proteins

Our bodies use protein to repair damaged tissues and cells, make enzymes and hormones, and maintain muscle, bones, skin, cartilage, and blood. Protein is an integral part to a healthy diet. There are various forms of protein, for example; quinoa, nuts, beans, eggs, Greek yogurt, cottage cheese, fish, and lean meats. It is best to add some sort of protein to at least one meal per day with small, protein-packed snacks in between exercise.

It is recommended that you not eat more protein than what can fit into the palm of your hand. Eating more than that can overload your kidneys and will take a lot longer to digest. Meats and other animal-based products *(dairy, eggs, and omega-3 fats)* are essential to your diet as they provide your body with much needed sulfur-containing amino acids which help you build more proteins.

When you have a sulfur deficiency, you are at higher risk of developing obesity, heart disease, Alzheimer's disease, and chronic fatigue. Sulfur aids the body in electron transport, synthesizing glutathione, regulates insulin production, and detoxification. It is when you start eating meats and animal products that have been highly processed, contain hormones, or the animal has been fed GMO corn or grain, that the meat is no longer beneficial for your body but destructive, causing inflammation. It is important to stick to organic, grass-fed/free range meats. I have discussed other healthy forms of meat later in this chapter.

Organic cottage cheese is great for lowering estrogen and oxygenating the blood and tissues, when combined with flaxseed oil. Eating ½ cup at breakfast with a little flaxseed oil will give you a huge boost for the rest of the day.

Whey protein shakes are great for quick snacks after exercise. Adding whey protein powder to your shake provides 25% of your body's calcium needs and 10% of your daily potassium. It is high in protein for rebuilding muscle and vitamin A for strengthening the immune system and overall gut health. I recommend *Axe Nutrition's Vanilla Whey Protein* which can be found on *store.draxe.com*.

Vitamins and Minerals

Your body needs many different vitamins and minerals to function and grow. Most of these important substances come from the food that you eat. Below are the most important vitamins and minerals that your body needs.

Vitamin E—

Vitamin E helps keep free radicals from entering the body and helps keep the immune system strong against bacteria and viruses. Foods such as almonds, peanuts, hazelnuts, sunflower seeds, spinach, broccoli, eggs, poultry, avocados, apricots, and olive oil are great sources in which to find high amounts of vitamin E. Combine the vitamin C and iron-rich foods for better absorption.

Vitamin C—

Vitamin C promotes healing and helps the body absorb iron. It also supports the creation of collagen and connective tissue. Citrus, red and green peppers, tomatoes, broccoli, guava, kale, kiwifruit, strawberries, and papaya are high in vitamin C. Don't forget to combine these foods with iron and vitamin E foods for better absorption.

Vitamin A—

Bone growth, vision, reproduction, cell function, and strengthened immune system are the roles that vitamin A plays in your body. Foods high in vitamin A include, sweet potato, carrots, kale, butternut squash, romaine lettuce, apricots, cantaloupe, sweet red peppers, tuna, mango, whole milk, and meat. Vitamin A works great when paired with vitamin C for the best results.

Iron—

Iron is a mineral that our bodies need to carry oxygen from our lungs to the rest of our bodies. It also helps our muscles store and use oxygen and is a component of hemoglobin. Squash, pumpkin seeds, chicken liver, mussels, clams, cashews, pine nuts, hazelnuts, almonds, beef and lamb, beans, lentils, bran, spinach, Swiss chard, and dark chocolate are full of iron. For the best absorption, combine these foods with the vitamin E and C foods above.

Vitamin D—

Vitamin D helps boost the immune system and aids the body in calcium absorption. A lack of vitamin D can lead to a bone disease called osteoporosis. Foods that contain vitamin D include egg yolk, saltwater fish, and mushrooms. Combine these vitamin D rich foods with the vitamin K foods for proper absorption.

It is becoming more of an issue amongst dancers, especially during the winter months, to have a vitamin D deficiency. Spending 20-30 minutes in the sun will help you absorb the amount of vitamin D you need for the day.

Vitamin K—

Vitamin K helps by making proteins for healthy bones and tissues as well as for blood clotting. Vitamin K can be found in Basil, kale, scallions, Brussels sprouts, chili powder, asparagus, fennel, leeks, okra, pickles, olive oil, and prunes. For proper absorption, make sure you are combining these foods with the vitamin D foods above.

B Vitamins—

All B vitamins use the food you eat to create energy and form red blood cells. The different B vitamins include B1 (thiamine), B2 (riboflavin), B3 (niacin), B5 (pantothenic acid), B6, B7 (biotin), B12, and folic acid.

B1 (thiamine) supports the function of the nervous system and the metabolism of carbohydrates. B2, B3, and B5 promote the metabolism of carbohydrates and fats. B6 supports protein metabolism and the creation of glycogen and glucose. The creation of red and white blood cells is supported by B6, B12, and folic acid. B12 also aids in gut, nerve, and tissue health.

Foods such as fish, poultry, beef and lamb, eggs, dairy, beans, peas, bran, sunflower seeds, macadamia nuts, acorn squash, asparagus, almonds, mushrooms, sesame seeds, spinach, avocado, sweet potato, pistachio nuts, prunes, bananas, lentils, mango, and oranges contain these B vitamins.

Calcium —

Calcium helps keep your teeth and bones strong, helps your muscles and blood vessels contract and expand, and secretes hormones and enzymes that send messages to the nervous system. Calcium rich foods include watercress, whole milk cheeses and yogurts, bok choy, okra, broccoli, green snap peas, almonds, sardines, buttermilk, whole milk, parsley, and molasses. Calcium works best when paired with magnesium.

Magnesium —

Supports protein synthesis and lowers inflammation. Magnesium can be found in spinach, collard greens, kale, Swiss chard, almonds, sunflower seeds, Brazil nuts, cashews, pine nuts, flaxseeds, pecans, mackerel, wild salmon, halibut, tuna, avocado, bananas, dark chocolate, and whole milk yogurt. For the best results and proper absorption, pair these foods with the calcium-rich foods above.

Zinc —

Found in cells throughout the body, zinc helps the immune system fight infection, bacteria, and viruses. Zinc also helps build proteins and DNA. Zinc can be found in beef and lamb, wheat germ, spinach, pumpkin seeds, squash seeds, cashews, dark chocolate, chicken, beans, and mushrooms.

Potassium —

Potassium is an electrolyte that supports muscle contractions and nerve impulse creation. Foods that contain potassium are oranges, whole milk, bananas, squash, fish, molasses, carrots, prunes, yogurt, kidney and lima beans, beets and beet greens, tomatoes, and sweet potatoes.

Fruits and Vegetables

Most fruits and vegetables are high in fiber, low in sodium and calories, and full of essential vitamins and minerals. Red fruits and vegetables can improve memory such as apples, raspberries, strawberries, cranberries, cherries, and beets. Some can even reduce stress; citrus, broccoli, papaya, mango, bell peppers, and kiwifruit for example.

Potassium helps regulate blood pressure and contraction of the muscles. Bananas, citrus fruits, cantaloupe, and kiwifruits are high in potassium.

Magnesium keeps bones strong, regulates blood pressure, keeps muscle and nerve function working properly, and lowers blood insulin levels. Apricots, avocados, and bananas are just a few foods that contain magnesium.

Simple and Complex Carbohydrates

Carbohydrates are basically made up of starch, sugar, and cellulose. Certain kinds of carbohydrates provide essential vitamins, minerals, antioxidants, and fiber. The best kind of carbohydrates to add into your diet are complex carbohydrates. Eventually, however, all types of carbohydrates turn into blood glucose, which is why you should limit the amount of carbohydrates you eat per day.

Complex carbohydrates are more natural and are much healthier for you, while simple carbohydrates are processed and broken down more. The complex carbohydrates contain all the vitamins and minerals that you need in your daily dietary intake. These types of carbohydrates take the form of oatmeal, quinoa, beans, buckwheat, and millet. They also have indigestible fibers that help with your gut health and even help with your bowel movements.

White bread, white rice, candy, sugar, and white baking flour are examples of simple carbohydrates. They are easily digested and absorbed quickly, causing a blood sugar spike and a sudden burst of energy that passes within a couple of hours. Simple carbohydrates have been processed so much that their natural fibers are gone or too broken down to benefit, giving them no importance to your body at all. Fruits and vegetables, all though considered simple carbohydrates, act as complex carbohydrates because of their fiber and protein content.

Choosing complex carbohydrates will help with lowering your risk of obesity, high cholesterol, digestive system diseases, and heart disease. An adult female should consume at least 25 grams of fiber a day. The next time you go shopping, try adding some of the following to your list:

Acorn squash	All-bran cereal	Amaranth	Barley	Black beans	Black-eyed peas
Buckwheat	Bulgur	Butternut squash	Garbanzo beans	Green peas	Kamut
Kidney beans	Lentils	Lima beans	Millet	Navy beans	Oat bran cereal
Oatmeal (not instant)	Oats	Parsnips	Pinto beans	Sweet potato	Quinoa
Brown, colored, or wild rice	Split peas	Sorghum	Spelt	Starchy vegetables	Whole grains (Ezekiel bread)

Metabolism

Metabolism is what controls your energy levels and determines how quickly your food is digested. It is a chemical reaction in the body's cells that converts the fuel from food into the energy you need to function properly throughout the day.

Higher metabolism may make you want to eat more because your body needs more energy to keep it going. The food that you are eating is being digested and turned into fuel so quickly that you need more in order to function. Because your body is using up all of its fuel so quickly and burning off all the calories with it, you will not necessarily gain weight.

The best way to make sure that you are staying healthy and maintaining a healthy weight is by eating a lot of fresh foods and healthy snacks. Snacks are great for keeping you feeling fuller, longer. Make sure you are not eating processed, sugary snacks as they can bring your energy levels down and can make you gain weight.

In order to keep your body in optimal condition to dance all day, you need constant refueling just like any other athlete. A stagnant person will not likely eat as much as an active one because they are not using up their energy resources.

When to Eat

Your performance schedule will determine when you will eat and what the portion sizes of your meals should be. If you have a long rehearsal before lunchtime with no breaks, make sure you eat a fairly large breakfast to compensate for that lost energy. Taking snacks with you is also a great idea if you start to feel hungry in the middle of class.

If you eat before your stomach starts growling, it helps to curb cravings for junk food. *"Hunger helps form neurological connections between taste and pleasure…by eating healthy snacks before cravings hit, you can weaken the link between junk food and addiction circuits in the brain."*

Breakfast is important because it is breaking your fast from dinner the night before. It starts your metabolism moving and gives you energy to start the day. Skipping breakfast can cause your body to be very sluggish and your thinking can be a little cloudy because your energy from the previous meal has been burned up.

Your body begins to slow down in the evening, burning less calories than during the day. Try to finish dinner at least 3 hours before you go to bed. You want to give your stomach enough time to digest what you have eaten before it becomes sedentary for the night. Midnight snacks might seem fun, but they are bad for your digestion.

Setting a meal plan and sticking to it allows for your body to be happy and healthy. Having small meals with snacks in between leaves one less likely to overeat. Even if you have a crazy schedule, it is important to not workout on an empty stomach. Make sure that you are continually fueling your body so that it does not go in to starvation mode. Avoid dancing on a full stomach as you could disrupt your digestion and get a stomach ache. It is best to wait 1-2 hours before any type of physical exertion.

The best thing you can do is eat something with complex carbohydrates (homemade granola bars, toast with bananas and almond butter, or oatmeal with berries) before your workout or dance class in order to provide your body with sufficient energy to perform. Afterward, make sure you are then eating a meal or snack that is packed with protein (boiled eggs, whey protein shake, or a turkey and spinach wrap) to rebuild the muscles.

If your schedule makes it too difficult to get nutritious meals on the table every night, consider *Sun Basket* (*sunbasket.com*) or other food delivery service. They allow you to choose your meals online which are then delivered, ready to assemble and cook in 30 minutes.

Another great way to eat your meals in the midst of a busy schedule is by packing bento boxes. Bento boxes allow you to bring your meals with you to eat on the ride to or from the studio. *Nom Nom Paleo* is a great resource for recipes and fun bento box lunch ideas. Some examples of what to pack inside:

Pre-Workout Box	Post-Workout Box
Granola & Yogurt	Turkey & Spinach Rolls
Berries or an Orange	Carrot Sticks
Homemade Granola Bars	Chicken Wings
Nuts & Dried Fruit	Cottage Cheese with Flax
Toast with Avocado	Bananas & Almond Butter
Sweet Potato with Coconut Butter	Vegetables with Quinoa

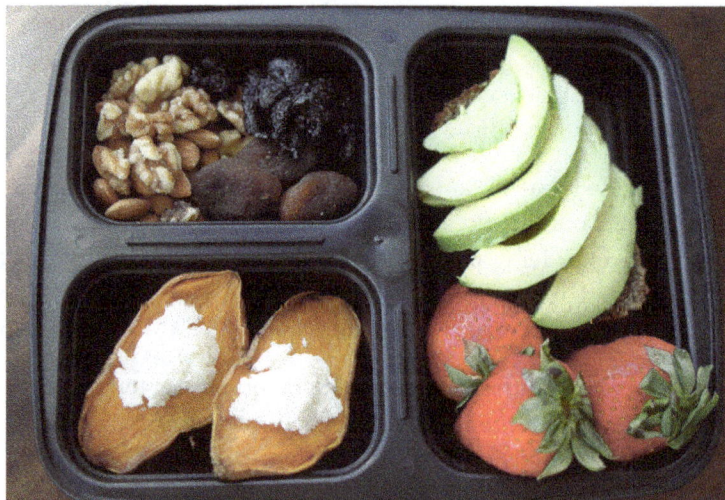

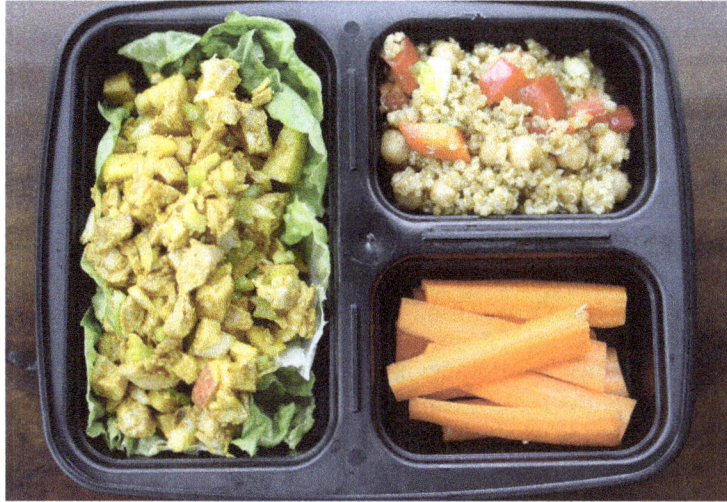

FOODS TO AVOID

GMO—

To get the most out of the foods that you buy, try to purchase non-GMO and/or organic. This is especially important when buying wheat, beans, vegetables, fruits, and grains. GMO (*genetically modified organisms*) foods are basically made in a laboratory. DNA from one species is transferred to another creating a completely new plant. Unfortunately, this creates genetic problems within the organism that can cause immediate as well as long term health issues.

A study done on rats that were fed GMO potatoes showed the females giving birth to stunted and/or sterile babies. Their organs were also beginning to fail as a result. GMOs are also horrible for the environment. Large amounts of pesticides and fungicides are used to keep the plants healthy. When it rains, the runoff from the plants can kill good insects, animals, and poison our water supply. Buying organically is the best way to stay healthy long term and you will know that you are helping your environment as well.

Non-Organically Raised Beef and Chicken—

When purchasing beef, you should ultimately look for organic grass-fed. Not only does buying organic help local meat producers, it is also healthier for the cows. The cows are normally raised in an open field where they are free to eat whatever they find in nature.

Look on the packaging to make sure the cows were raised without antibiotics or hormones. You also want to make sure there are no additives such as color or flavor as they may contain MSG. Grass-fed beef has a richer amount of omega-3 fatty acids and tastes so much better!

Chicken—

Living in an area where chickens are raised by the truck-load, I know how poor their living conditions can be. When purchasing chicken, look for USDA organic certified. This means that the chickens have been raised 100% organically from egg to plate.

Most chickens are raised with antibiotics and hormones and their feed can sometimes contain pesticides and herbicides. The antibiotics given to chickens can also create strains of bacteria that are resistant to those antibiotics, causing more of a potential for human disease.

Free range chickens are happier and healthier than chickens raised in cramped chicken houses. If the chicken is barely able to move, it can "stunt" the meat growth giving it little to no health value or taste. Buying organically will be much healthier and tastier.

RECOMMENDED DIETARY INTAKE FOR DANCERS

It is important to know exactly how much your body needs of certain nutrients, vitamins, and minerals for proper, healthy meal planning. Below is a chart outlining the main nutrients that your body needs on a daily basis. All the measurements are requirements for all persons aged 4 and older.

Total Fat	65 g	Healthy fats loaded with omega-3 and omega-9 to support brain health
Cholesterol	300 mg	Helps the body properly break down Vitamin D, regulates hormones, and promotes proper brain function
Sodium	2400 mg	An electrolyte that is needed to promote blood and fluid regulation

Potassium	3500 mg	Works to enhance muscular strength, metabolism, and water balance
Total Carbohydrate	240-300 g	Complex carbohydrates provide energy and healthy weight control
Fiber	25 g	Blood sugar control, healthy bowels, and weight management
Protein	50-98 g	Can reduce the risk of heart diseases and helps the body's cells and tissues function properly
Vitamin A	5000 IU	A powerful antioxidant that boosts the immune system and prevents infection and disease
Vitamin C	60 mg	Boosts immunity, lowers blood pressure, and prevents free radicals from entering the blood stream
Calcium	1000 mg	Aids in bone and dental health
Iron	18 mg	Metabolizes proteins and aids in the production of hemoglobin and red blood cells

The reason why it is important to know what your daily requirements should be, is so that you can supplement any areas that you are lacking in with whole food sourced vitamin supplements or by simply adjusting your diet. Supplements that are from whole food sources are healthier because your body will recognize and absorb them better than conventional supplements. The amounts listed are the total amounts that you need from both food and supplements per day as an active person. To prevent deficiencies in certain areas, the RDA has put together this list of measurements of these particular vitamins and minerals.

SMART SHOPPING

Buying and eating organically can be a little expensive. Fortunately, there are ways to help stay within your budget and still eat organically. The first step is removing the junk food and extra snacks that you can live without. You really do not need that tub of ice cream, soda, or that bag of potato chips, do you? Probably not. Removing those "extra" items will help bring your grocery bill way down.

Another great way to save a ton of money, is by making things at home. Baked goods, homemade potato chips, popcorn popped at home, and homemade granola bars are great (and easy) ways to save money on snack foods. I will provide you with a few easy recipes at the end of this chapter.

"Dirty Dozen"

If you want to shop organically but are on a tight budget, try sticking to the "dirty dozen" for organic buys. These fruits and vegetables tend to absorb more toxins than most and should be bought organically. If you can't find them organic, peel them and wash them thoroughly.

Apples	Peaches	Nectarines	Strawberries	Grapes	Celery
Spinach	Sweet bell peppers	Cucumbers	Cherry tomatoes	Imported snap peas	Potatoes

The safest vegetables and fruits to eat non-organically include:

Onions	Avocados	Sweet corn	Pineapples	Mango
Asparagus	Kiwi	Cabbage	Eggplant	Cantaloupe
Grapefruit	Sweet potatoes	Bananas	Sweet peas	Watermelon

Eat Your Greens

I know a lot of people do not exactly love to eat green vegetables, but they are extremely good for you. They are high in vitamins and minerals such as vitamins A, E, C, and K, iron, magnesium, calcium, folic acid, carotenoids, omega 3 fatty acids, and fiber.

Daily intake of green vegetables will help prevent cell damage, risk of cancer and heart disease, helps keep your digestive system regular, helps you lose weight, and they are low in carbohydrates and glycemic levels. Try to purchase most of your greens organically.

The best greens to eat include:

Watercress	Chinese cabbage	Chard	Beet greens	Spinach
Chicory	Leaf lettuce	Parsley	Romaine	Collard greens

You can even grow your own bean sprouts. They are an excellent source of vitamins B, C, B1, B6, K, and A. They are also rich in iron, magnesium, phosphorus, calcium, potassium, omega 3 fatty acids, and manganese. Eating a handful a day can increase oxygen levels in your blood stream and boosts the immune system as well as aid in digestion, losing weight, and they are great for your skin!

I recommend mung bean, sunflower, and broccoli sprouts. They taste great and are extremely good for you. You can eat them raw, in a stir-fry, or you can juice them. Growing them is easy and will save you money.

- *First, wash out a jar*
- *Rinse off the freshly-dried mung beans (or seeds)*
- *Pour the beans into the jar (only about ¼ inch)*
- *Cover the beans with filtered water for 8-10 hours*
- *Drain the beans and cover with muslin or cheese cloth*
- *Keep the beans in a cool, dry place for 2-3 days*
- *Make sure you rinse the beans once/day to keep them clean and free from any mold*

Meats

Of course, meat can make a huge hole in your wallet when buying organically. That is why you make the meat that you buy stretch as long as you can. Eating small amounts of meat at meals will allow for leftovers and will save you money. Go for the highest quality meat no matter how expensive and make it stretch by alternating meat with other protein sources.

Oils

Olive oil and coconut oil are probably the best oils to use when cooking or baking. Olive oil is great for dressings, spaghetti, and on top of baked chicken, while coconut oil is great for stir-fry, baked goods, and fried foods.

When buying olive and/or coconut oil, I recommend extra virgin. Extra virgin is nothing but the natural, pressed oil from the olive or coconut. Because it is nothing but pure oil, they tend to be more flavorful and fruity. All oils should be purchased in their purest form to maintain the health benefits and taste.

MENU PLANNING TIPS

When planning your menu for the week make sure you are keeping your meals small and sporadic. Half of your plate should be non-starchy vegetables (carrots, broccoli, Brussels sprouts, etc.), one quarter of your plate should be grains or starchy vegetables (sweet potato, squash, brown rice, etc.), and one quarter protein (chicken, beef, egg, beans, etc.). Fruits and dairy should be eaten in moderation and fats can be found in oils, fish, avocados, etc.

Dancers and athletes need constant refueling to maintain their optimal endurance and performance levels. Having snacks in between meals allows for constant replenishment of lost protein and enzymes. The best meal plan to follow to maintain a constant refueling without over-eating, is by eating three small meals (breakfast, lunch, and dinner) with snacks in between.

Snacks

I love making my own snacks because I can tailor them to my taste preferences and cravings. To save money and keep your belly full, here are a few of my favorite snack recipes.

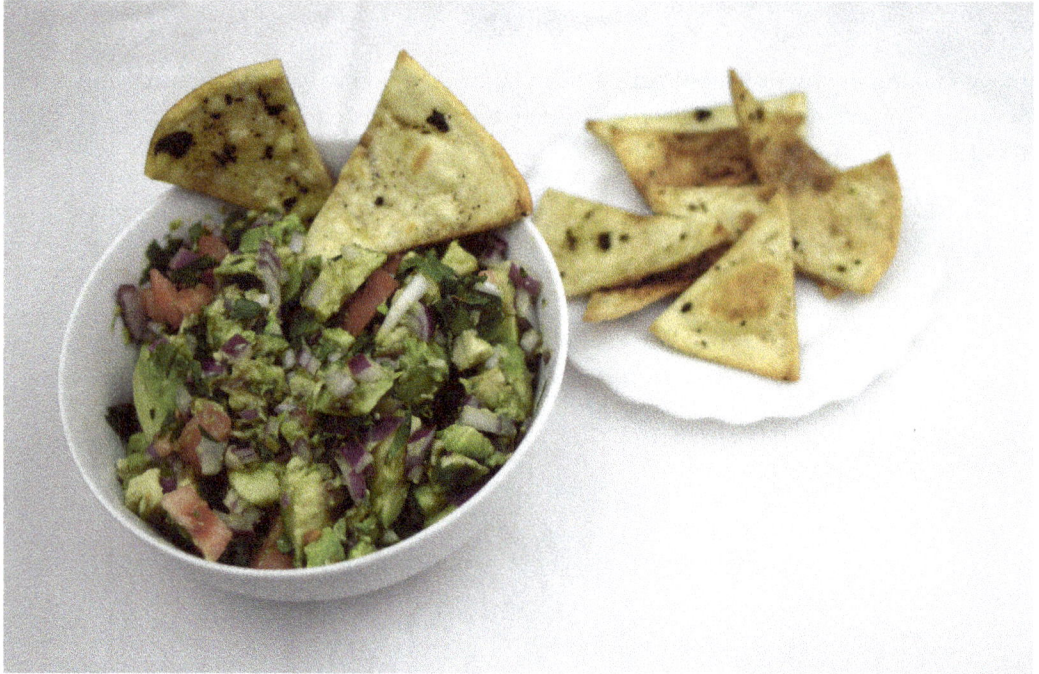

Chunky Guacamole with Homemade Pita Chips

Guacamole Ingredients:

- 2 avocados – peeled, pitted, and chopped
- ½ lime, juiced
- ½ teaspoon sea salt
- ½ cup onion
- 3 tablespoons fresh cilantro, chopped
- 1 plum tomato, chopped
- 1 teaspoon minced garlic

Pita Chips Ingredients:

- 4 pita bread pockets
- ¼ cup olive oil
- ¼ teaspoon black pepper
- ¼ teaspoon dried basil
- ¼ teaspoon garlic salt

Instructions:

Put all the guacamole ingredients in a bowl and toss together. For smoother guacamole, put everything into a food processor and pulse for 2-3 minutes.

For the pita chips, preheat the oven to 400 degrees. Cut each pita pocket into 8 triangles and place on a cookie sheet. In a small bowl, combine the oil, pepper, salt, and basil. Brush the triangles with the oil mixture and place in the oven for about 6 minutes, or until lightly browned.

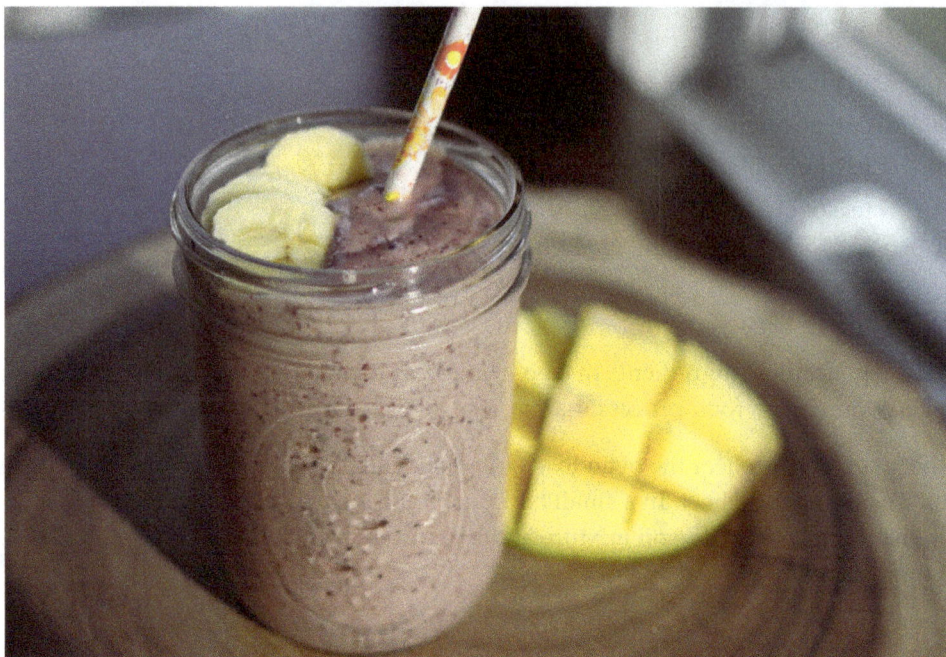

All-Day Energizer

Ingredients:

- ½ mango
- ½ banana
- Handful blueberries
- 4 oz. water
- 1 tablespoon or scoop protein powder
- 2 tablespoons yogurt
- 1 teaspoon or scoop green powder supplement

Instructions:

Blend all the ingredients in a blender and enjoy!

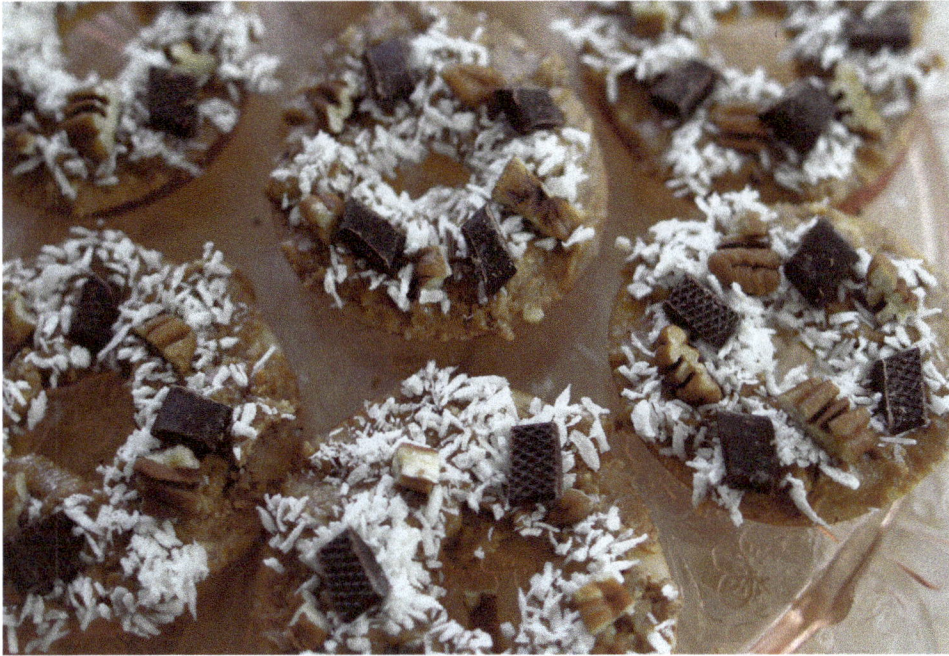

Apple Cookies

Ingredients:

- 1 apple, washed
- Almond butter
- Shredded coconut
- Chocolate chips or chocolate chunks
- Chopped pecans or walnuts
- Cinnamon (optional)

Instructions:

Start by sliced the whole apple into large "cookie" slices. Using a small paring knife, gently cut out the core or use a small, round cookie cutter. Spread the almond butter over each slice. You can either sprinkle the coconut on or pour some on a small plate and tap the apples into the coconut. Top with chopped nuts and chocolate chips. Sprinkle with cinnamon and enjoy!

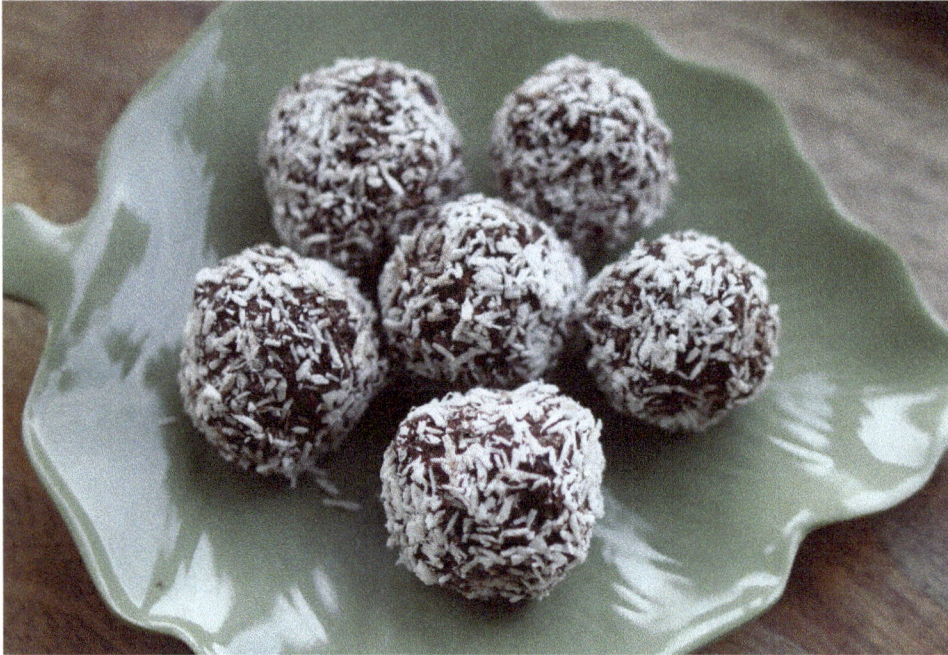

Cocoa Bites

Ingredients:

- 2 cups whole pitted dates
- 1 cup unsweetened shredded coconut
- 1 cup whole almonds
- ¼ cup plus 2 tablespoons unsweetened cocoa powder
- Enough water to make a paste

Instructions:

Process the dates, coconut, almonds, and cocoa powder in a food processor until the nuts are finely chopped. Add the water and pulse until the mixture forms a rough paste. Shape heaping tablespoons into balls and roll in chopped nuts or coconut. Keep refrigerated for up a week.

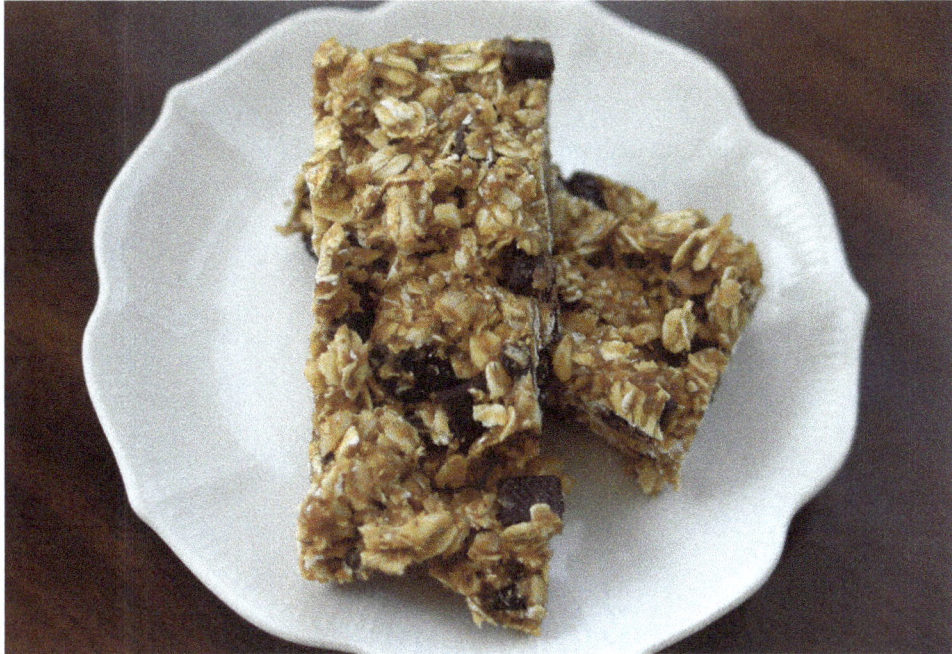

Homemade Granola Bars

Ingredients:

- 1 cup pitted dates
- ¼ cup honey or maple syrup
- ¼ cup creamy natural peanut butter or almond butter
- 1 cup roasted almonds, roughly chopped
- 1 ½ cups rolled oats
- Chocolate chips, dried fruit, nuts (optional)

Instructions:

Process the dates in a food processor until slightly doughy. Place the oats, almonds, and dates together in a mixing bowl and set aside. Warm the honey and peanut butter in a small saucepan over low heat until smooth.

Pour the mixture over the oat mixture and stir until fully incorporated. Add in any extra ingredients such as the chocolate chips or dried fruit. Do not be afraid to use your hands to get everything incorporated.

Transfer to a lined 8×8 baking dish pressing down firmly until flattened. Place in the freezer for 15-20 minutes, or until firm. Cut into granola bars and wrap in parchment paper or eat. These can be stored in an airtight container for up to a week.

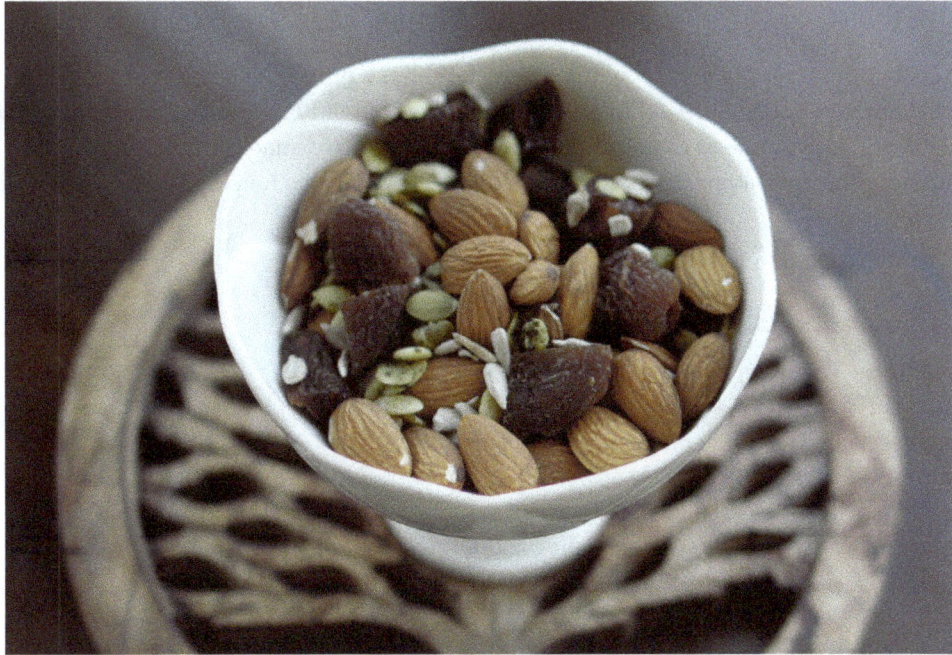

Snack Mix

Ingredients:

- Pumpkin seeds
- Almonds
- Sunflower seeds
- Dried apricots, cut into quarters

Instructions:

Toss all ingredients together and enjoy. Can keep up to a month in a sealed container. You can substitute any of these ingredients with cranberries, chocolate chips, walnuts, pecans, Brazil nuts, raisins, or any other dried fruit or nut that you would enjoy.

Sample Menu

To make your menu planning a whole lot easier, I have put together a list of food groups and the amount you should eat in one day. As I have already mentioned many times, to save money, I recommend eating three small meals and two snacks in between throughout the day rather than three large ones. This will also help space out your food a little more.

Vegetables – *5 servings a day*
Fruits – *1-2 servings a day*
Meats – *enough to fit into the palm of your hand per meal*
Dairy – *1-2 cups a day (limit the amount of milk you drink)*
Carbohydrates – *240-300 grams of complex carbohydrates a day*
Sugars – *6 teaspoons a day (not including fruits)*

To help you with your meal planning, I have provided a sample daily menu, weekly menu, and a food journal that you can be inspired by and fill out on your own.

"One of the very nicest things about life is the way we must regularly stop whatever it is we are doing and devote our attention to eating." –Luciano Pavarotti

BREAKFAST	SNACK	LUNCH	SNACK	DINNER	DESERT
½ c. cottage cheese with pineapple and flaxseed	½ c. guacamole with garlic	Sesame stir-fried chicken salad with tomatoes, cucumbers, dark greens, and bell peppers	8 oz. whey protein shake with greens	Radish and fennel salad with bean sprouts and pepitas	Papaya with lime and honey
Soft-boiled egg with a slice of Ezekiel toast or Turkey sausage	Plantain chips, Terra chips, homemade pita chips, or rice crackers	Sprinkle of pumpkin seeds	OR	½ c. hummus on the side or Salmon	
Matcha green tea or Ginseng tea			Handful of raw nuts (almonds, walnuts, or pecans)		

BREAKFAST	SNACK	LUNCH	SNACK	DINNER	DESERT

SAMPLE WEEKLY MENU (recipes from *Stress Less Cooking by Deidra Howard*)

Meal	Monday	Tuesday	Wednesday	Thursday	Friday	Saturday	Sunday
Breakfast	Rainbow frittata with ginseng tea	Hot millet cereal with steamed apples and Turkey sausage	Breakfast egg bagel with green tea	Green immune juice with poached egg and bacon	Mexican eggs	On-the-go muffins with Matcha tea	Gingerbread pancakes with homemade applesauce
Snack	Stress relief snack mix	Cleansing vegetable juice with whey protein	Handful of nuts (almonds, cashews, walnuts)	Fruit kabobs with yogurt	Power snack	Chocolate banana sandwich treats	Nut and seed mix
Lunch	Chicken pesto sandwich with veggie sticks	Superfood vegetable pasta	Salmon with Indian spices and curried quinoa	Thai chicken soup with spinach salad	Indian lamb stew with Moroccan beet salad	Spinach and tuna salad	Roast beef salad
Snack	Watermelon and raspberry salad	Power snack	Apple oat cake	Cleansing vegetable juice	Crisp rice squares	Stress relief snack mix	Chewy granola bars
Dinner	Black bean and shitake soup with Japanese ginger salad	Hummus and vegetable sandwich with curried carrot soup	Quinoa vegetable salad	Cubin black bean soup with corn bread	Greek pita salad	Fresh salad with miso dressing and some pumpkin seeds	Hot borscht with kale and onion stir-fry
Dessert	4 oz. square of dark chocolate	Quick fruit sorbet			Guilt-free pumpkin cake with cinnamon icing		Papaya with lime and honey

Meal	Monday	Tuesday	Wednesday	Thursday	Friday	Saturday	Sunday
Breakfast							
Snack							
Lunch							
Snack							
Dinner							
Dessert							

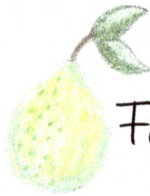

Food Journal

TODAY I ATE—

NEW FOODS THAT I TRIED:
_____
_____
_____

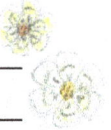

MY FAVORITE FOODS:
_____
_____
_____

FOODS I PREFER NOT TO EAT AGAIN:
_____
_____
_____

Water Log

CHAPTER SIX

Eating Disorders

DEALING WITH THE MIRROR

Appearance is everything in this day and age. We focus so much effort on how we look instead of how we feel on the inside. Nobody wants to be an outsider; thus, we try to fit in by making ourselves more fashionable, thinner, or we change our personalities all together.

As dancers, there is a specific body type that many dance companies and studios look for when advancing to a professional. Unfortunately, this puts a lot of pressure on those of us who are built bigger or more muscular. Not everyone is going to look thin and lanky. A great example is Misty Copeland. She is defying the odds when it comes to being a professional ballerina. Her chest is not a size A and her legs and arms are super muscular, yet she is still able to do everything a dancer like Polina Semionova or Natalia Osipova can do.

Your body was built a certain way for a certain reason. Making it into something it is not is just simply wrong. Self-image is obviously a huge problem among many people, especially young girls. They will look in the mirror and see something (or many somethings) that they simply do not like about themselves. When you go through puberty, your body changes a lot. This can cause a few self-image issues with certain girls.

If your self-image continues to get worse, it can turn into a serious health issue. When we do not accept who we are, we are in conflict with ourselves. We need to be in agreement with ourselves otherwise, we become disconnected with who we really are and this can lead to depression and fabricated, people-pleasing personalities.

To maintain a happy and healthy lifestyle, you need to love yourself. Everyone has minor imperfections, but that is what makes you beautiful and unique. I am built more muscular than the other "typical" ballerinas, but that doesn't hold me back because I love to dance. I just accepted that I need to work a little extra to maintain a healthy weight for my body type.

Quite a few dancers feel that they must go to the extreme when it comes to fitting in with the "perfect" ballerina mold. This can oftentimes lead to eating disorders that will ultimately damage their bodies and cause many illnesses. Dancers, or just young ladies in general, can succumb to an eating disorder much easier if they already struggle with depression, a sense of loneliness, or if they feel a lack of control within their environment.

Coming into acceptance is the first thing you need to do to become a healthier person. If you do not accept your body and who you are, how do you expect others to accept you? Believe me, people will know when you accept yourself. You will exude confidence that will inspire others. They will end up enjoying your company and will want to be around you because you accept who you are. You are beautiful just the way God made you and nobody can tell you otherwise.

Don't look in the mirror and think of all the things you would like to change. Instead, look at yourself and say, "I am beautiful! Today I choose to be beautiful inside and out." This can be difficult for some dancers because they are dancing in front of a mirror all throughout class, picking out every wrong movement they are doing or noticing the differences between classmates and themselves. Look at your own attributes that you enjoy and appreciate about yourself and use them to their full potential.

"Dancers are perfectionists, and we often focus on what we're doing wrong instead of all the beautiful things we're doing. Every day I tell myself, 'I am enough.' I don't have to prove myself to anyone, and I'm already putting in 110 percent, so I don't have to push myself any harder. I am enough." **–Alicia Graf Mock** (Natural Health Magazine, March/April 2014)

Stay positive and maintain your focus on working to stay healthy. Eat a proper diet and create a fun exercise program that makes you happy. The exercise will provide your brain with "happy" hormones; endorphins, that can lift your mood and energy levels. They will give you a great boost for the day.

Having poor self-image can sometimes cause disorders such as anorexia nervosa, bulimia nervosa, and binge eating disorder. These can become very dangerous illnesses that need to be stopped before they become detrimental.

There are ways to prevent them from happening, but if you are already struggling with one of these disorders, I hope to give you a few words of encouragement in this chapter. You can get through this! I believe in you! You now need to believe in yourself.

RECOGNIZING THE SIGNS

It is important to recognize the signs of an eating disorder as a friend of someone starting one or if you are falling into an eating disorder yourself. This way you can catch it earlier on and put it to a stop. Keep in mind that dancers tend to be three times more at risk than the average person.

The most common eating disorders are Anorexia, Bulimia, and Binge eating. They all have different signs but all can cause the same amount of damage to your physical and emotional health.

Anorexia Nervosa

The most common of all eating disorders, anorexia nervosa is when a person starves themselves to lose weight. The lack of appetite that a person with anorexia feels is often induced by nervousness and is controlled by an intense fear of gaining weight. When they start to feel that they are no longer in control of their weight, anorexia can develop to keep that weight off.

Common signs of anorexia include weight loss, feeling cold, avoidance of food or avoidance of settings where food is present, odd eating habits, fatigue, use of laxatives, binge eating, withdrawal, perfectionism, mood swings, and low self-esteem.

When someone has anorexia, their body starts to go into hibernation and enters starvation mode. This protects the body as long as it possibly can until it succumbs to death. The long-term effects include, blood sugar drops, bones become very brittle and weak, muscles lose their mass, they begin to experience hair loss, organs fail, menstrual periods slow or stop, and their hair and nails become dry and cracked.

Having a copper deficiency can cause your body to shut off appetite causing you to eat less and fall into an anorexic state. I recommend that you get a hair analysis to test your copper levels.

Bulimia Nervosa

The next common eating disorder is bulimia. Usually a person with bulimia overeats and then purges when they are finished in order to get rid of it. Like anorexia, bulimia is meant to help the person lose weight.

The signs include tooth decay, a frequent sore throat, binging, overuse of laxatives, mood swings, sores on the hands or knuckles, frequent bathroom trips, dehydration, irregular heartbeat, extreme exercise, constant self-criticism, and eating in secret. People who struggle with bulimia long-term are at a higher risk for throat cancer and a damaged digestive system.

Binge Eating Disorder

Binge eating disorder is when someone is constantly overeating food. It often feels uncontrolled and is spaced out during the day. Eating large amounts of food very quickly, eating all alone, depression, anxiety, dieting without any significant weight loss, self-criticism, feeling guilty after eating, and hoarding of food are signs that someone is struggling with binge eating.

Those that struggle with it have a higher risk of high blood pressure, panic attacks, problems with their digestion, stroke, depression, heart disease, and Type 2 diabetes.

TREATMENTS

Recovery from any of these three eating disorders can take time and a lot of patience.

Treatment usually involves first, admitting that you have a problem, then you should consult your doctor or a specialist to make sure that you are not struggling with other health issues and so that they can put you on a long-term plan.

It is easiest to catch the eating disorder before it becomes an obsession. This can often be just as difficult as seeking treatment once it has gone too far. The most important thing you need to do first is to admit to yourself and others that you are struggling. Once you have that out of the way, it will be easier for your family and friends to support you and encourage you as you try and break the habits that you have fallen in to.

Try and stay away from influences, whether they be people, circumstances, or things, that can encourage self-criticism or self-loathing. Always be thinking about yourself in a positive way. Loving yourself is the best thing you can do to avoid falling into an eating disorder.

Being prepared as a young woman for the changes that will inevitably happen during puberty will prevent any surprises. Your body will change and get a little curvier but it should not be seen as a bad change. Expect the change and learn to accept it early on.

Talk to someone about struggles you are going through. A friend, sister, or your mom are great support systems to have behind your back when you are going through a tough time. Talking to someone close and being honest can often resolve a lot of issues all on its own.

I hope that I have encouraged and inspired you in this chapter. I believe in you! You are beautiful and loved. You are amazing just the way you are.

"Be yourself. If you water yourself down to please people or to fit in or to not offend anyone, you lose the power, the passion, the freedom and the joy of being uniquely you. It's much easier to love yourself when you are being yourself." –Dan Coppersmith

---

The Power of Positivity

THE GOOD THINGS ABOUT TODAY:

_____

_____

_____

WHAT I HOPE TO ACCOMPLISH TOMORROW:

_____

_____

_____

PEOPLE THAT MADE ME HAPPY TODAY:

_____

_____

_____

THINGS THAT MADE ME HAPPY TODAY:

_____

_____

_____

MY HAPPY QUOTES

All About Me

I AM HAPPY BECAUSE: _____

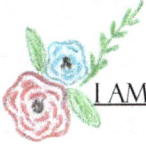

_____

_____

I AM BEAUTIFUL BECAUSE: _____

_____

_____

_____

WHAT MAKES ME STAND OUT? _____

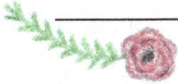

_____

_____

_____

MY FAVORITE PART(S) ABOUT MYSELF IS: _____

_____

_____

_____

"The best and most beautiful things in the world cannot be seen or even touched – they must be felt with the heart." –Helen Keller

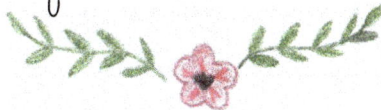

CHAPTER SEVEN

Staying Healthy Year-Round

Getting sick can cause a huge impediment when it comes to dance, especially during the winter months. Missing classes leaves you falling behind and out of shape. Maintaining a strong immune system throughout the year ensures that the cold and flu seasons will not affect you as bad and allergies will be a thing of the past.

First of all, you want to make sure you are not pushing your body too hard. If you feel like you are getting tired too quickly or sore too often, it might be time for you to take a break or lessen your time in class. If your body is stressed out, physically and mentally, it can lower your immune system and make you more susceptible to colds and the flu. Balance your emotional stress levels by doing things that you enjoy (*Check out chapter 8 for stress reducing suggestions*).

Make sure you wash your hands each time you come home from the studio. You never know what germs you pick up on the barre. Before you wash your hands, try not to touch your face as germs can be spread very easily through your eyes, nose, and mouth.

Drink plenty of water! Staying hydrated is extremely important to keeping your immune system in proper working order. Water helps your body flush out toxins that can build up in your body. If you will remember, we discussed the benefits of staying hydrated and how much water you should drink in the *Health and Nutrition* chapter.

Make sure you are getting enough sleep. The average adult needs up to 8-9 hours of sleep (10 p.m. – 6 a.m.) per night, while the average adolescent needs about 10-11 hours of sleep (10 p.m. – 8 a.m.) per night to stay healthy. For dancers, or any athlete, it is important that they sleep a reasonable amount of time every night. Your muscles need rest from the hard work they have done during the day. Sleeping will help your body heal and recover faster. If you feel tired, it is probably your body telling you that you need some sleep.

BUILDING A STRONG IMMUNE SYSTEM

Possibly the most important step to building and maintaining a strong immune system is by eating well year-round. You want to make sure that you are eating foods that are high in vitamins, antioxidants, enzymes, and minerals. Grass-fed organic milk, whey protein and/or collagen, kefir (a cultured, enzyme-rich food full of microorganisms that balance your immune system), fermented pickles, organic miso, sauerkraut, olives, blueberries, mushrooms, and lots of vegetables are great examples of immune-strengthening foods. The fermented foods support gut health by bringing in good bacteria that defend against pathogens and aid in the production of antibodies.

Organic, whole milk contains beneficial bacteria that supports the immune system and can reduce allergies. It is also a great source of vitamin A and zinc, two very important vitamins that your body needs. Whey protein is great when you cannot find raw or organic milk. It contains beta glucans and immunoglobulins which help with your body's natural detoxification processes.

If you are dairy-free, try coconut milk as a substitute. Coconut milk kefir is also a great way to still get your vitamins and minerals while avoiding dairy. There are many other dairy-free options including coconut milk yogurt, almond milk, and cashew milk. Avoid soy milk whenever possible (soy is discussed in more detail in the *Foods to Avoid* section of this chapter).

All berries are high in antioxidants and are low glycemic. Portobello, porcini, and crimini mushrooms are rich in protein, fiber, vitamin C, B vitamins, calcium, and other minerals that strengthen the immune system.

Organic extra-virgin coconut oil is excellent for your thyroid and metabolism. It is rich in lauric acid which strengthens your immune system. This can be taken as a supplement as well if you would prefer.

The richest source of caffeic acid and apigenin, two very potent compounds that aid in immune response, is propolis. Propolis is a resin found in the bee hives surrounding the honey.

Chlorella (a freshwater algae) contains chlorophyll that helps you produce more oxygen, cleanses your blood, and promotes the growth and repair of tissues. It also binds to toxins and carries them out, protecting your immune system against illness.

Wheatgrass—

Wheatgrass has become a popular little shot of energy among the health conscious. It is packed with vitamins A, C, E, K, and B, as well as iron, calcium, magnesium, selenium, chlorophyll, amino acids, and bioflavonoids. Wheatgrass is normally drunk in 2 oz. shots or it can be frozen into cubes and put in smoothies. You can also purchase wheatgrass powder for smoothies or supplements.

Many people who drink wheatgrass shots on a regular basis experience an increase in energy, weight loss, increase in athletic endurance, increase in immune system, lower blood pressure, decrease in susceptibility to infection, lower cholesterol, normal blood sugar levels, and an increase in blood flow throughout the body increasing the oxygen levels in cells.

Spices and Teas

Certain spices also offer amazing immune boosting properties and some can even act as expectorants. These spices include cinnamon, cloves, turmeric, garlic, licorice, black pepper, anise, cardamom, thyme, bay leaf, and oregano. Most of these spices also have anti-inflammatory properties which makes them great for when you get sick.

Green tea, Matcha, and Tulsi tea are rich in antioxidants. Matcha has 17 times the antioxidants of wild blueberries and seven times more than dark chocolate. Tulsi tea can help with memory, heart health, vision, along with supporting the immune system. Herbal teas such as astragalus tea, lemongrass tea, elderberry tea, and nettle leaf tea are also great for immune support. I shared my favorite immune boosting tea in chapter 2 that I recommend that you try.

Ginseng is a great anti-inflammatory and virus suppressing root that can be steeped in a tea or put into a soup. Chicory is an expectorant and great when steeped into a tea with a little manuka honey. Manuka honey is full of immune boosting vitamins and mincrals.

Echinacea helps boost the white blood cell count, thus activating the immune system. It is best taken at the first sign of a cold. Turmeric can be taken in warm milk for anti-inflammatory benefits and it will also help you sleep. Add a little manuka honey to add a touch of sweetness.

Chamomile is great for easing stress and anxiety, settling the stomach, and promoting restful sleep. Adding a little honey and some lemon is great for sore throats.

All of these herbs can be found on *MountainRoseHerbs.com* and the manuka honey can be found in your local health food store or online on *Amazon.com*.

Essential Oils

Eucalyptus oil or tea tree oil diffused helps loosen phlegm that can build up in the lungs and soothes blocked airways. They are also anti-bacterial and anti-fungal which helps remove any cold and flu germs that may be in the air.

Lemon oil is calming, anti-sceptic, disinfectant, detoxifying, and anti-fungal. Diffusing lemon essential oil can help reduce fever, treat insomnia, and decrease the risk of infection.

Lavender oil can enhance circulation, lower anxiety levels, ease respiration, and relieve pain when applied directly to the skin or diffused into the air.

Bergamot oil, grapefruit oil, and tangerine oil are all great for stress and anxiety. They work as anti-depressants by increasing hormone secretion and blood circulation.

There are two ways to administer essential oils-

- By using an essential oil diffuser (6-7 drops in the water)
- Or by adding 6-7 drops of essential oil to a carrier oil (coconut oil, almond oil, or olive oil) and rubbing it on the bottoms of your feet at night.

Foods to Avoid

Try and avoid soy products as they can lower your immune system response and damage your thymus (a gland where immune cells mature). If you would like more information on soy and its damaging effects, I recommend that you visit Dr. Mercola's website. He shares studies and many facts on soy that will help you understand why I do not recommend it as a helpful food product.

Limit your sugar intake. Too much can lower your immune system making you more susceptible to getting sick. Try adding fresh fruits to your diet instead and use natural sweeteners such as honey, molasses, and maple syrup as they do not raise your blood glucose levels as high as regular sugar does. These natural sweeteners also contain minerals that are essential to your diet. Finally, try to avoid artificial colors, flavors, and preservatives.

COLD AND FLU SEASON

Even though cold and flu season seems a little daunting, it *is* possible to avoid getting sick as long as you keep your immune system strong. Maintaining a healthy, vitamin-filled diet is key to avoiding the flu. If you start to feel a cold creeping up, take extra vitamin C such as *Airborne* to give you a boost. Garlic and ginger are great for kicking a cold. Try making a soup with lots of fresh garlic and ginger and maybe add some cayenne or habanero and your cold will be gone in no time.

> *When you start to feel sick, crush one clove of garlic and spread on a slice of bread with butter on it. The raw garlic contains allicin which helps fight infection. If you are feeling really bad, the garlic bread can be eaten up to 4 times a day for a week or until you start to feel better. You can also add some raw honey or butter for added benefit.*

Spend time out in the sun to get your daily dose of vitamin D. As I have previously mentioned, vitamin D is essential to a strong immune system. Because we are stuck inside during the colder months, it is important to supplement your diet with foods or supplements that are rich in vitamin D such as cod liver oil, herring, rainbow trout, salmon, sardines, and eggs. If you have allergies or these do not appeal to you, there are excellent supplements available that provide the same benefits. *Green Pasture Products Blue Ice Cod Liver Oil* has a variety of different oils including blend of many important fish oils. You can find these online.

A hot water bottle and castor oil can be used for lymph drainage, increasing circulation, reducing inflammation, and easing cramps and digestive issues. If you feel that you are starting to get sick and your lymph nodes are a little clogged and swollen, placing a hot water bottle on them will help get the lymph fluid flowing.

> *Rub some castor oil into the area, place a flannel cloth over it, cover with plastic wrap, and then top it with the hot water bottle. Leave it on for at least 20 minutes.*

Apple cider vinegar added to water can ease nausea and stomach illness. Likewise, a tea made of crushed and boiled cumin seeds is also very effective in relieving nausea.

1 Tbsp. of honey and ¼ tsp. of cinnamon can be taken daily for a week to strengthen the immune system and ease a sore throat.

For sore throats and sinus infections, gargle salt water twice a day until you feel better. Warm water with lemon, raw honey and onion will also help with a sore throat.

To clear up nasal passages, try soaking your feet in a bath of hot water and add 10-15 drops of peppermint or eucalyptus essential oil. This foot bath will also help in relieving headaches.

Another option for clearing up nasal passages is by soaking your feet in a hot bath with the essential oils for about 10 minutes. Afterward, dry off your feet and put on cotton socks that have been soaked in cold water. Layer some dry, wool socks over top and then go to bed.

RECOVERING QUICKLY

Instead of using over-the-counter drugs that can contain corn syrup, dyes, and artificial flavors, I recommend using alternative ways of relieving cold and flu symptoms.

Oscillococcinum is the best homeopathic flu reducer that I have used. When taken at the first sign of the flu, your symptoms will disappear within a couple of days. You can purchase it at *Walgreens* or any store that sells cold medicine. It is a homeopathic and must be taken 20 minutes before or after food to work properly. Make sure you take it as often as the package directs or your symptoms will not go away as quickly.

Airborne is great for colds and works pretty quickly. I usually take it whenever I have been around people who are sick and whenever I am starting to feel cold coming on. Airborne offers effervescent tablets that you can drop into your water or chewables that you can just pop in your mouth.

Chestal is my favorite product for coughs and sore throats. It tastes like honey and is the only cough syrup that works almost immediately and lasts for a long time. Chestal also works to clear up nasal congestion and sneezing.

Smart Silver can be gargled and swallowed for sinus injections and sore throats. It is anti-microbial and works fast to relieve injections and illness. Take ¼ cup 3 times a day until symptoms subside.

You can find Smart Silver online at *smartsilver.com, Amazon.com,* and in some Health Food stores.

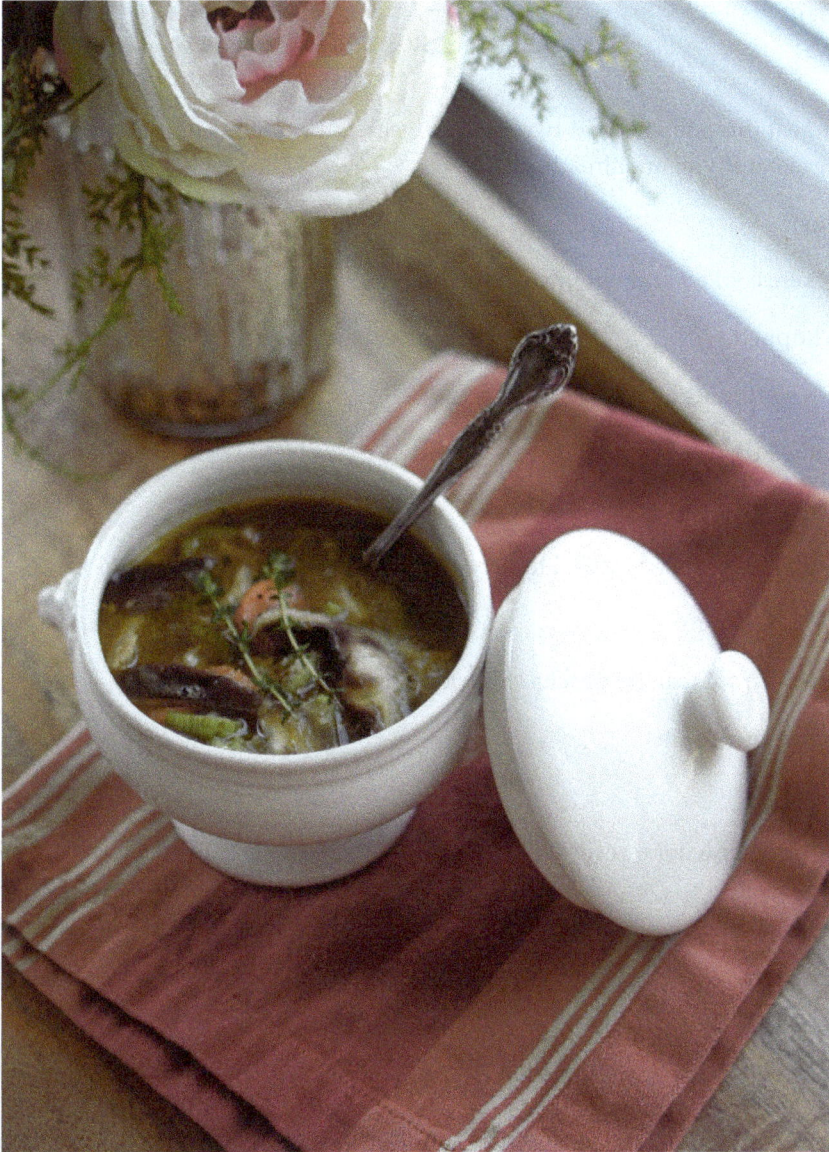

Immune Support Soup

It is best to eat this soup at least two times a week to keep your immune system strong or to recover faster if you are already sick.

Ingredients:

1 cup chicken, cooked and cut into bite-sized pieces

1 onion, chopped

3 stalks of celery, sliced

2 carrots, sliced

2 parsnips, sliced

½ bulb fresh garlic, smashed and minced

1 inch fresh ginger, minced

¼ cup burdock root (can be purchased dried), ground

8 oz. shitake mushrooms

2 Tbsp. olive oil

1 Tbsp. ginseng powder or crushed, fresh root

4 cups bone broth

2 bay leaves

1 tsp. thyme

Directions:

Sauté the vegetables in a pot with the oil until the onions are translucent and the garlic is aromatic. Pour in the broth and add the spices and chicken. Bring to a simmer for 20 minutes. Serve into bowls and enjoy!

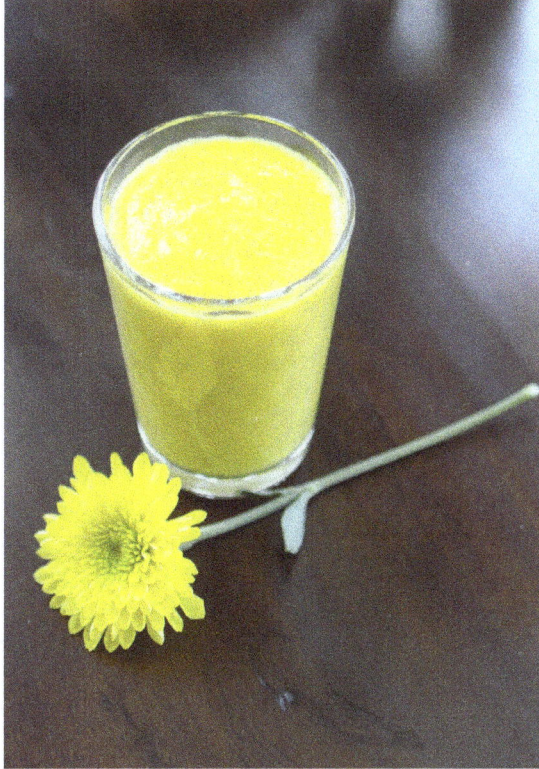

Super Immune Juice

Ingredients:

1 whole lemon

1 peeled orange or grapefruit

1 Tbsp. Manuka honey

Enough water to blend

Directions:

Place all the ingredients into a blender and puree until smooth.

For a super immune booster, add in ½ tsp. cayenne, 2 cloves of garlic, and ½ tsp. horseradish. You can drink this tonic daily when you start to feel sick. If you are really sick, the tonic can be drunk up to three times a day.

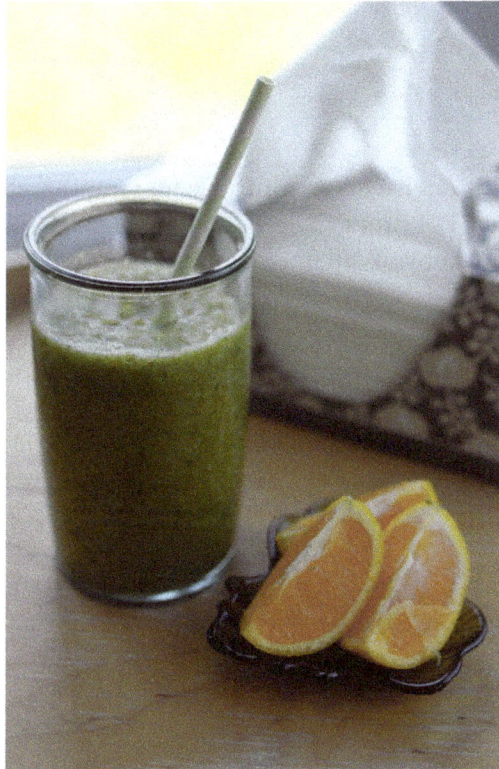

Cold and Flu Juice

Ingredients:

1 pear

2 stalks celery

1 lemon or lime

2 carrots

1 nectarine

1 cup honeydew melon

1 orange

1 inch ginger

1 handful kale or spinach

Directions:

Place all the ingredients through a juicer or in a blender until smooth. If you are using a blender, add a little water (1/4 cup) to help everything blend easier. Drink within 12 hours to get the best results or you can freeze it into popsicles.

SEASONAL ALLERGIES

Allergies can come in many different forms, the most common being sensitivity to mold and pollen. Coughing, sneezing, itchy eyes, stuffy and runny nose, and sometimes sore throat can be signs that you are suffering from seasonal allergies. Most of the time allergies are caused by a weakened immune system. Because your immune system is weak, you are most susceptible to mold, pollen, pet dander, and other forms of allergy-causing particles.

80% of your immune system is located in the gut. Maintaining healthy gut flora and good bacteria will help lower your chance of being affected by allergies. Eating foods that are rich in probiotics and foods that are fermented can help build gut flora and good bacteria. I mentioned a few of these foods earlier in this chapter in the *Building a Strong Immune System* section.

Vitamin D is also essential to building a strong immune system. Spend at least 20 minutes in the sun every day to get the amount of vitamin D your body needs. Raw honey contains propolis, which as we discussed earlier is great for building a healthy immune system. Add some honey to your tea, baked goods, or just enjoy a teaspoon full for a quick boost. Manuka honey is also a great choice for its immune boosting properties.

To support lymph drainage, try drinking 8 ounces of water with a tablespoon of apple cider vinegar.

It is best to not tax your immune system by eating too much sugar, GMO foods, artificial dyes and preservatives, and foods that contain MSG. You also want to make sure you are getting enough sleep and keeping your stress levels to a minimum (the damaging effects of stress is discussed in more detail in chapter 8).

Allergy Medication

Just like with cold and flu medications, allergy medications can contain artificial colors and flavors which can weaken your immune system even more. Allergy medication can also have a multitude of side effects and the relief felt can be short-lived. It can tear down the body creating a cycle of allergies and increasing your risk of long-term cognitive impairment.

The best, and most natural ways, to improve allergy symptoms is by eating well and by maintaining your daily intake of important vitamins and minerals.

A homeopathic called, *Allergy* by *Heel BHI*, is my favorite way to ease symptoms caused by seasonal allergies. This homeopathic can be found online and in some Natural Food Stores.

You can also use a saline nasal spray to clear up mucus and to remove any allergens in the nose.

I hope that this information helps you the next time you are struck with a cold, the flu, or just plain allergies. Remember to maintain a healthy diet as this will be the foundation on which your immune system will be based.

PART THREE

Happy Dancer

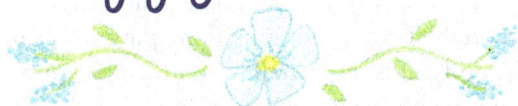

CHAPTER EIGHT

Stress Managment

As dancers, we are always busy learning choreography, staying fit while at home, and

making sure we eat healthy. This can cause a lot of stress and anxiety for some, making it easier for them to succumb to prolonged stress and even burnout. Stress is also one of the worst offenders when it comes to low immune system and illness. Keeping your stress levels to a minimum is extremely important to maintaining a healthy lifestyle.

STRESS AND ITS EFFECT ON YOUR BODY

Stress is not always avoidable, however, there are plenty of ways to reduce the amount

of stress that you let into your life daily. Fear, anxiety, and even unresolved anger can cause a cascading effect on the body eventually damaging the adrenals, gut, and the repair capabilities of the body. It is important to be at peace (for more information I recommend reading *Stress Less Cooking by Deidra Howard*).

As I mentioned in chapter 1, stress is the enemy when it comes to staying healthy. You will remember that when you are stressed, cortisol and adrenaline are released as your body goes into "fight or flight" mode. When you are constantly stressed, cortisol is regularly released into your blood stream. Too much cortisol will decrease the function of your adrenal glands.

Adrenal glands are what control certain hormones to keep the body functioning properly. When your adrenal glands are depleted, you can start to get headaches and muscle aches due to hypersensitivity in the brain and nerves. Chronic fatigue, little to no sleep, weight gain, unhealthy food cravings, susceptibility to infections and illnesses, sensitive intestinal tract, anxiety, and depression are also symptoms of adrenal fatigue.

High cortisol levels on a long-term basis can also impair cognitive function, suppress the thyroid gland, decrease bone density and muscle tissue, raise blood pressure, increase the risk of hypoglycemia, slowed healing, and lower the immune system.

I know that the dance year can be very stressful on parents who have to drive to and from dance classes. On my website, adancersdiarybook.com, I have offered a special section in which parents of dancers can share their tips and questions on how to maintain a stress-free environment for themselves and their dancer.

AVOIDING BURNOUT

Burnout is what happens when you are in a state of emotional, mental, and physical exhaustion. If you are constantly working in a stressful or high-pressure environment or if you are putting too many expectations on yourself, you can end up being burnt out and exhausted.

Having burnout and being overly stressed are two very different things. Unlike stress, burnout is when emotions are blunted and there is a lack of motivation that can easily lead to depression. The main reason depression sets in is because you are no longer feeling in control of your emotions or environment and your mental and physical exhaustion starts to make you feel ineffective.

Signs of burnout include chronic fatigue, insomnia, forgetfulness, impaired concentration, lack of attention, chest pain, heart palpitations, shortness of breath, gastrointestinal pain, dizziness, fainting, headaches, lower immune system, loss of appetite, anxiety, depression, and increased irritability.

Burnout is an extreme level of stress that usually comes from working too hard with little to no recovery time. It is important that you not push yourself beyond what you know you can handle. Overtraining is the most common cause of athletic burnout. Your performance will begin to decline and you will then start to lose interest in the sport or art that you previously loved. This can oftentimes be misdiagnosed as clinical depression.

Your main motivation when it comes to dance is to do it because it is something that you love. When that motivation changes into a need for approval or recognition within your community or team, you tend to be more susceptible to burning out due to the stress of over-achieving.

JUST BREATHE AND BE HAPPY

Happiness can be different for different people. Some people are happy reading outside on a warm, sunny day in a hammock for hours, while others enjoy going to a bowling alley with friends.

To avoid burn out and high stress levels, it is important to find ways to keep your stress levels down to a minimum. This can be hard when there is so much to do every day. There are many simple activities that you can do to help you relax and enjoy yourself.

Being Happy

Try planning a night out with your friends to laugh and have fun. Laughing is truly the best medicine! You can also watch a comedy or play a fun game. Laughing relaxes your muscles, boosts the immune system by decreasing stress hormones, releases endorphins, increases blood flow throughout your body, eases anxiety, and improves mood.

"Your sense of humor is one of the most powerful tools you have to make certain that your daily mood and emotional state support good health." **–Paul E. McGhee, Ph.D.**

Gardening is also a great way to reduce stress. Start a garden in your backyard or have a few potted plants in your home. It is a great way to get your exercise with the repetitive movements such as pulling weeds and digging.

Digging in the dirt can actually increase your ability to metabolize serotonin, the hormone that controls cognitive function and elevates mood. Not only that, you are also getting the vitamin D from the sun that your body needs to maintain a healthy immune system.

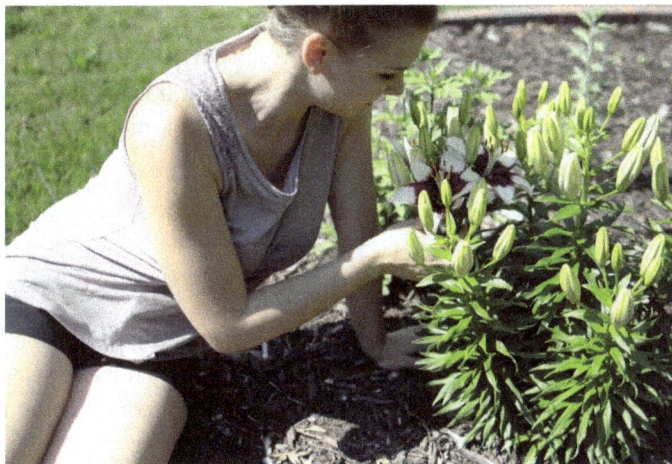

If gardening is not for you, then just spending time outside in the fresh air can do the trick. Take a walk or simply sit on your front step and read a good book. Going to the beach and putting your feet in the sand is also extremely relaxing. It provides you with necessary minerals and great exercise!

Another great way to reduce stress levels is drawing. Drawing and coloring, allows you to be creative and distracts you from whatever was bothering you. Now that adult coloring books are becoming so popular, I recommend that everyone have one for particularly stressful days. Journaling is also a great way to alleviate stress in some people. Writing helps you put things into perspective.

Listening to music is my favorite stress reliever. I love classical music but when I really need a pick-me-up, sometimes I will listen to either Broadway or the best 80s hits. They make me want to dance and that will often remove all stress. Pick the music you especially love and put it all together in its own playlist. The next time you are stressed, listen to that music and dance around your room.

Relaxing in a hot bath is my next favorite way to ease stress levels. I love to light candles, put essential oils and Epsom salts in the water, and watch a movie or listen to music. When I am having a really stressful day, or have been extra tense, I give myself a mini massage on my neck and shoulders.

Another way to alleviate tension in your muscles is by tightening them for 3 seconds while holding your breath. Letting your breath out, release your muscles completely. Repeat this 12-14 times to release tension.

Did you know that giving someone a hug can reduce cortisol levels? A hug that lasts over twenty seconds can lower blood pressure, reduce cortisol levels, alleviate tension, releases endorphins, and boost the immune system. I think it is amazing how just one hug can do all of that. The next time you feel stressed, give someone a hug and see if you feel different.

Breathing

Take deep breaths when you start to feel anxiety. Fill your lungs completely and mentally force your muscles to relax. Breathe in through your nose for two seconds (1-1000, 2-1000) and breathe out through your mouth for four seconds using the same counting method. Do this 12 times to exercise your lungs.

To make sure you are filling your lungs, imagine you are first filling your stomach, then your chest, and lastly, your head. Let the air out through your mouth slowly. Breathing deep helps you to relax and provides your brain with lots of fresh oxygen.

Just remember to stay calm and positive throughout your day. It will make all the difference when you start your day with the right attitude.

THE IMPORTANCE OF GETTING ENOUGH SLEEP

Getting enough sleep during the night is crucial to staying healthy. Proper amounts of sleep can help you lose unwanted fat and is important for maintaining healthy energy levels during the day.

Melatonin is produced while you are sleeping and is taken to your bloodstream. The pineal gland in your brain produces it. During the day, it is usually inactive. Melatonin helps to fight cancer and is what makes you feel tired at night. If not enough melatonin is made, the more at risk you are of developing tumors.

When you start to feel sleepy, that is usually your body telling you to go to sleep. It is important that you not ever skip or shorten your sleep times. You also want to make sure you are not exercising past 4 o'clock as this can cause insomnia.

Avoid watching T.V. or using the computer at least an hour before falling asleep. The light they give off tricks your brain into thinking it is daytime. This will decrease your melatonin levels making is harder to fall or even stay asleep. Make sure any electrical devices are at least 3 feet away to avoid any interference with your sleep.

It is best to sleep in complete darkness and with cooler temperatures. The ideal temperature for comfortable sleep is between 68 and 70 degrees Fahrenheit.

If you have a hard time falling asleep at night, try taking a hot bath or shower 1-2 hours before bedtime. Reading a good book and drinking a calming tea, such as chamomile, is also a great way to relax just before bed.

Insomnia can be caused by a magnesium deficiency. Make sure you are eating some of these magnesium rich foods to avoid a deficiency in this important mineral.

Spinach	Swiss Chard	Beans
Almonds	Pumpkin Seeds	Sunflower Seeds
Sesame Seeds	Avocado	Kale

Getting enough sleep at night will help you heal faster, decrease your risk of injury, boost your mood and immune system, promote clearer thinking, controlled weight, and improves memory. Healthy adults should get 8-9 hours of sleep every night, while adolescents need 10 or more hours of sleep each night.

As tempting as it is to stay up late watching movies and eating midnight snacks, it is not healthy and can take a toll on your body. Of course, occasionally, it is fun to stay up late, just do not make it a habit. Once it is a habit, it is very hard to break. I promise that if you get a good night's sleep, you will feel 100% better in the morning.

Fun Quotes and Pick-Me-Ups

"You are responsible for your own happiness. If you expect others to make you happy, chances are you'll always end up disappointed." **–Unknown**

"Laugh as much as you breathe and love as long as you live." **–Unknown**

"I love it when someone's laugh is funnier than the joke." **–Unknown**

"I like people who make me laugh. I honestly think that laughing is the thing I like most. It cures a multitude of ills. It's probably the most important thing in a person." **–Audrey Hepburn**

25 Things to be Happy About

1.
2.
3.
4.
5.
6.
7.
8.
9.
10.
11.
12.
13.
14.
15.
16.
17.
18.
19.
20.
21.
22.
23.
24.
25.

My Favorite Quotes

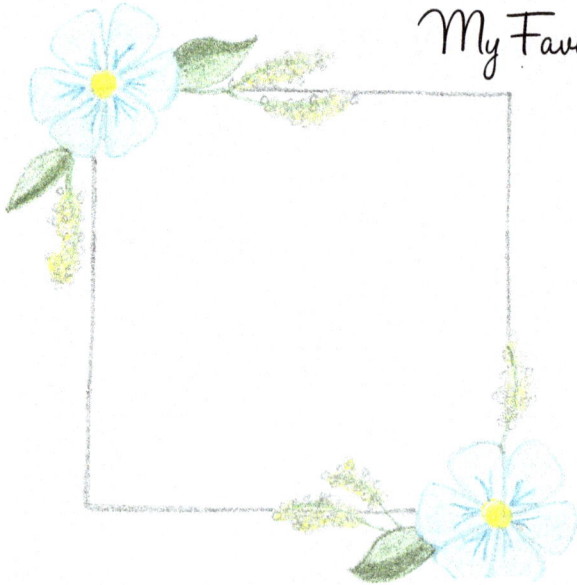

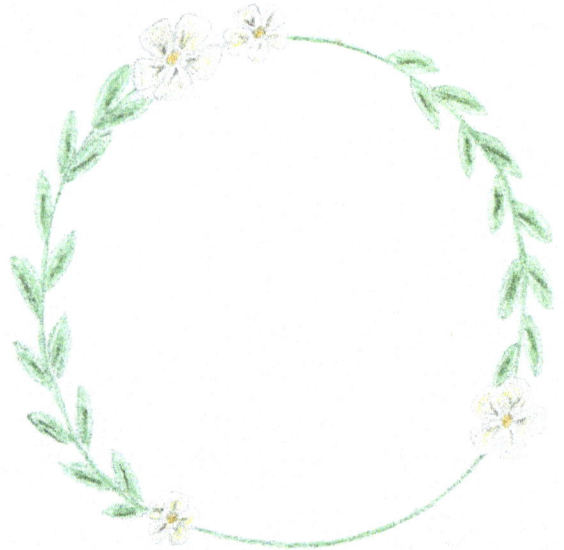

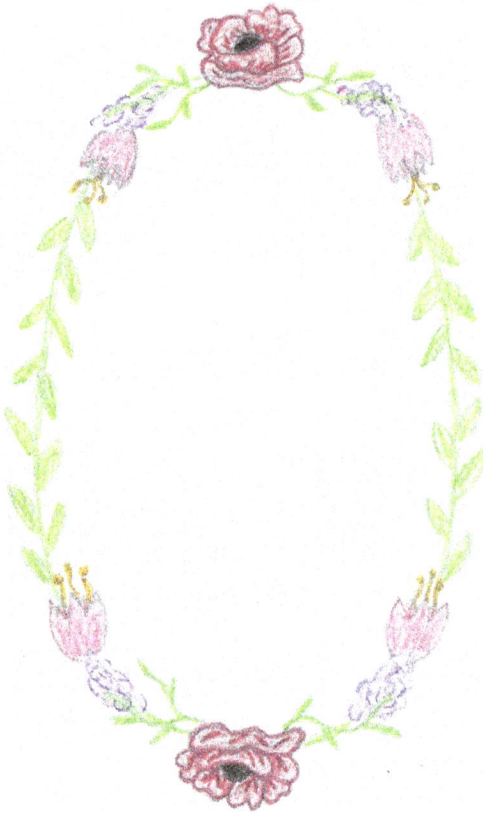

Tasks That Need Completed

_____ / _____ / _____

MOST IMPORTANT TASK FOR TODAY:

◊ _____

NEXT IMPORTANT TASK FOR TODAY:

◊ _____

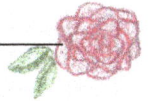

ADDITIONAL TASKS:

◊ _____
◊ _____
◊ _____
◊ _____

NOTES

"Focus on Being Productive Instead of Busy" - Tim Ferris

Today's Inspiration

_____ / _____ / _____

TODAY I AM THANKFUL FOR:

_____

_____

_____

TODAY IS GOING TO AMAZING BECAUSE:

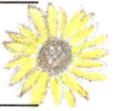

_____

_____

_____

TODAY I WOULD LIKE TO IMPROVE ON:

_____

_____

_____

THE QUOTE THAT INSPIRES ME TODAY IS:

_____

_____

_____

TODAY I LEARNED:

_____

_____

_____

"Dear old world ... You are very lovely and I am glad to be alive in you." -Anne of Green Gables

My Week

THIS WEEK I AM EXCITED FOR: _____
_____
_____

MY MAIN FOCUS FOR THIS WEEK: EXERCISES I WOULD LIKE TO TRY:
_____   _____
_____   _____
_____   _____

THINGS I HOPE TO ACCOMPLISH THIS WEEK: FOODS I WOULD LIKE TO TRY:
_____   _____
_____   _____
_____   _____
_____   _____

NOTES

CHAPTER NINE

Getting Ready for the Big Night

Dancers spend copious amounts of time learning their routines in order to commit it

to muscle memory. At that point your body just moves to the music and there is not much thought when it comes to the choreography. However, there are still things that can go wrong such as stage fright and slight costume malfunctions. In this chapter I share the best ways to remove these obstacles for a smooth, continuous performance.

RECITAL PREP

Being properly prepared is one of the most important ways to ease nervousness about

your upcoming performance. Getting everything you need packed ahead of time allows you to take your time getting ready for your recital, instead of rushing around last minute. Make sure your costumes are completely protected in a garment bag along with all the accessories that go with them. Pin the accessories to the matching costume with a safety pin to make sure nothing gets mixed up.

Double check your dance bag to make sure you have all the items you need to perform and warm up with. You also want to make sure that you have first aid items just in case and extra makeup, hairspray, and baby wipes for little messes. A small sewing kit is also a great idea in case you need to fix your costume or Pointe shoes.

Arrive early to your performance location so that you know where you should be and to get settled in. Hang up your costumes and put your dance bag in an easily accessible area. Check your makeup and put on any hair accessories and jewelry. Arriving early also allows you to spend time warming up and going over your choreography.

We will discuss more items that you can pack in your dance bag at the end of this chapter. I have also created a checklist to help you keep track of everything.

WARMING UP

Warming up before you go on stage is important for avoiding any injuries while dancing. When your muscles are cold, they are more prone to strains and pulls so it is important that you not go on stage until your muscles are ready. Find a hallway or dressing room with enough space to do some warm-up exercises and stretches. Exercises such as plies, tendus, developpes, grande battements, échappés, and changements are great choices to get your muscles warm and ready to stretch and perform.

To increase your flexibility, perform stretches such as a lunge stretch, quad stretch, port de bras, calf stretch, and the splits. Do not hold these stretches too long as they may lengthen your muscles making it harder for them to perform properly.

If your muscles are tight due to tension, use a foam roller or tennis ball to massage them out. Releasing the fascia will help keep you limber for your performance. You can also do a simple self-massage on your neck and shoulders to ease nervousness and to help you relax (see Chapter 3).

STAGE FRIGHT REMEDIES

The recital season is both the most exciting and also the most nerve-wracking time of the year. You have been rehearsing for what feels like ages, and now you finally get to wear your costumes and do your makeup and hair. The comradery back stage with all the laughing, joking, and eating snacks is so much fun. Then you line up, ready to step onto the stage.

Almost every performer gets stage fright, especially when they are waiting in the wings about to perform. To ease some of the butterflies, make sure you are fully prepared to walk out onto that stage. Warm-up in the hallway or dressing room to make sure your muscles are ready to go, and do not forget to stretch. Stretching and deep breathing is great for releasing stress and tension.

Eating snacks such as bananas and dried apricots are a great before a performance because the potassium that they contain can help lower blood pressure. Yogurt is full of probiotics that reduce the activity in the emotional part of the brain, helping to decrease anxiety and worry. Stay away from alcohol and caffeine as they can intensify your anxiety.

When I get nervous, I usually take a homeopathic called, *Gelsemium Sempervirens*. It works quickly and efficiently at relieving stage fright and apprehension. This homeopathic can be found in Natural Foods stores and online.

Another great way to both clear your mind and calm your nerves is by drinking a cup of chrysanthemum tea. Add a little manuka honey to give some sweetness.

MAKEUP AND HAIR

Your costume and choreography are perfected and ready to be shown off. The last step is making sure your makeup and hair are just as beautiful as your dancing. Stage lighting can be harsh and can wash you out if you are not properly prepared.

Makeup

Some dance studios require that you wear certain colors on your eyes, lips, and face. Make sure that you are checking with your teachers to make sure you are following any guidelines that they may have.

Once you have that out of the way, it is important to know how to apply your makeup so that you are not blending into the background. Here are some great tips for stage makeup.

First, wash your face to remove any oils that will cause your makeup to streak. It will also provide a clean canvas for you to work on.

Apply your foundation with a brush or sponge starting in the middle of your face, working outward. Choose a color that is slightly warmer than your natural skin tone so that you do not wash out under the stage lighting. Blend the foundation all the way up to your hairline, and below your chin and jawline. If you need extra coverage, use a light concealer and blend it out evenly.

To make your face stand out more on stage, use bronzer and blush to contour your face. Apply your blush on the apples of your cheeks, following it all the way to your temples. Bronzer can be applied to the hollow of your cheeks, between your eyebrows in a "V" pattern, down the center of your nose and along your jawline.

Highlighter can also be used to enhance the contours of your face. Apply light highlighter on the cheeks, chin, forehead, and underneath your eyebrows.

For your eyes, some dance studios require certain colors for eyeshadow. Make sure you are complying with what your teacher has asked that you wear. Pinks, creams and light browns can be used on the eyes if not specified by your teacher. Apply a light color on the whole lid and define the crease with a slightly darker shade.

Thinly line your upper lashes with a black or dark-brown eyeliner. For the bottom lashes, you can either line the water line or directly under the lashes with the same color liner. You can also do a slight cat-eye by flicking up the outer adage of your eyeliner.

Fill in your eyebrows with a similar color as your hair, following the natural curve of your brows. You can also use an eyebrow gel to keep the hair in place throughout your performance.

Apply mascara by gently moving the brush side-to-side to ensure you cover each lash. False lashes can also be used to enhance the thickness and length of your lashes.

Choose your lipstick based on the character you are portraying, and what your fellow dancers are wearing. Red, pink and peach are the most common lipstick choices for dance recitals. First, line your lips with a lip-liner that is close in color to your lipstick, and fill it in. Apply the lipstick on top.

Powder your face to set everything and to remove any extra shine.

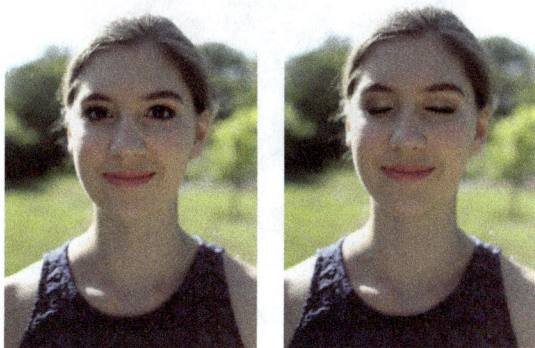

Make sure you wash all of the makeup off after the performance to prevent breakouts. Use a makeup remover or gentle cleanser all over your face. Coconut oil is great for removing waterproof makeup and it also moisturizes your skin. Toner or exfoliant will help remove any excess makeup left behind. Do not forget to moisturize your face after you have finished.

Hair

As with your makeup, be very clear on what your teachers expect you to do with your hair. Most teachers are pretty flexible with hair styles, as long as all your hair is out of your face. Adding braids or twists to your classic ballet bun allows for creativity and elegance. To prevent hair breakage, use U shaped pins and elastics that do not have a metal piece on them.

French-braided bun:

Start by French-braiding two braids, coming closer together as you move down. Secure them with elastics. Gently pull the hair out a little to make the braids look thicker. Wrap one braid into a bun, pinning as you go. Repeat with the other braid. Spray thoroughly with hairspray.

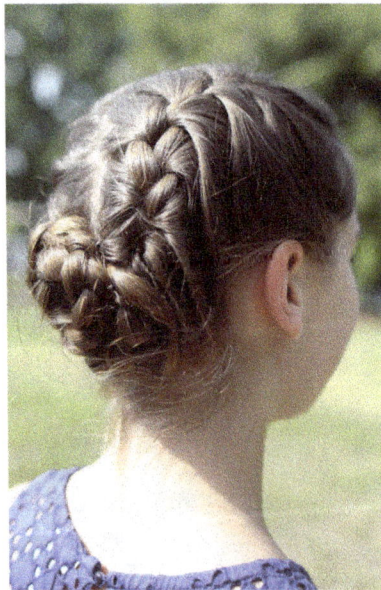

Twisty bun:

Starting on the right side, take two small sections of hair. Twist them around each other once, adding a little more hair to the bottom strand. Continue this until you reach the back of your head and secure with bobby pins. Repeat the twist on the other side and secure. Take all your hair and start twisting it into a ballet bun. Use a hairnet for extra security and spray with hairspray.

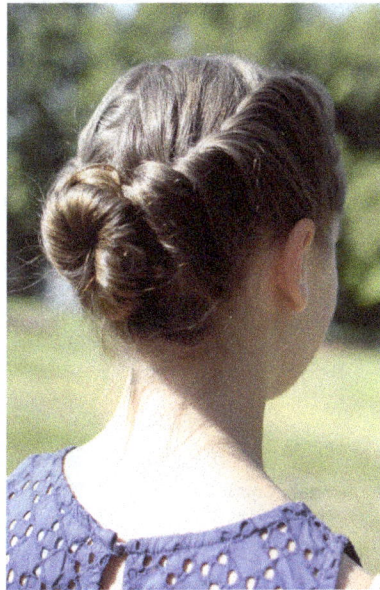

Ballet bun:

Brush all your hair into a high ponytail. Separate the ponytail into two sections and start twisting the first section. Wrap it around the elastic, twisting and pinning as you go. Repeat this process with the other section of hair. For extra security, wrap a hairnet around the bun and secure with bobby pins. Spray with hairspray.

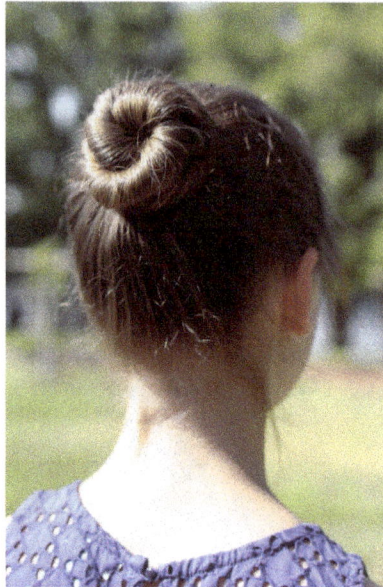

RECITAL ESSENTIALS

Because you want to be prepared for all circumstances during a performance, it is important to pack a few extra things that you may not usually need during class. Double check to make sure you have all the shoes you need to dance in, an extra pair of tight in case one pair tears, and warm-up items such as leg warmers and a sweater.

For injuries that may occur, pack a mini first aid kit with band aids (both regular and blister). Baby wipes are great for any spills or makeup malfunctions. Pain relievers and sore muscle rub can also be packed in case of emergencies.

Hang your costumes on hangers in garment bags to keep them safe. Safety pin all of your matching accessories to each costume to simplify the changing process between dances. A mini sewing kit and extra safety pins are also very important for any rips or lose jewels and ribbons.

Pack extra makeup, hairspray, bobby pins, elastics, and a brush or comb in a separate bag for touch-ups. Water and snacks are also important to pack to keep hydrated and just in case you get hungry in between acts.

Finally, bringing music or a book with you is great to keep you focused and occupied when you are waiting back stage. However, it is always more fun to goof off with your friends.

I have provided a checklist that should help you with your packing process at the end of this chapter. I find that having a checklist helps me keep track of what I need to bring with me.

I wish you the best of luck with your next performance!

Recital Checklist

Extra Tights
Shoes
Costumes and Accessories
Warm-Up Sweater, Leg Warmers, and/or shorts
Makeup
Compact Mirror
Bobby Pins and Hair Ties
Hairspray
Brush or Comb
Bandages (regular and blister)
Mini Sewing Kit
Wipes
Pain Relievers and Muscle Rub
Deodorant
Water
Snacks

PART FOUR

Beautiful Dancer

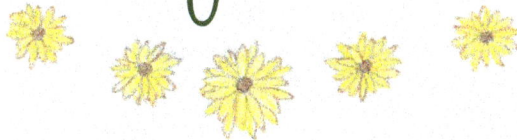

CHAPTER TEN

Taking Care of Your Dancing Feet

As ballet dancers, we all know how important it is to keep our bodies in good condition. Our feet are no exception. In this chapter, we will discuss the various toe and foot ailments that affect dancers as well as ways to strengthen and take care of our lovely dancing feet.

HOW TO PREVENT BUNIONS

Bunions are caused by inflammation of the joint in the big toe. This inflammation causes an abnormal enlargement of the joint at the base of the toe. The first metatarsal is displaced and can move into or under the other four metatarsals causing the bone to project. The good news is that most bunions are treatable without surgery.

Some symptoms of a bunion include:

- *Pain in and/or around the big toe joint*
- *Limited mobility*
- *An enlargement of the base of the metatarsal*

One way to prevent bunions is by using toe spacers. Toe spacers allow a space in between the big toe and second toe preventing some of the 'squishing' especially when *en pointe*. You can also do some simple tension exercises that will strengthen the muscles that keep the toes in place.

Put a thick rubber band on both of your big toes. Stand with your feet hip-width apart. Without moving your feet, start moving your big toes away from each other. Repeat four times.

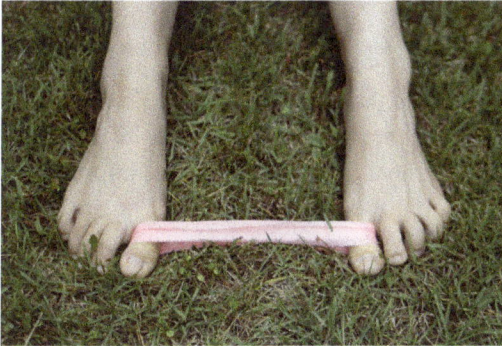
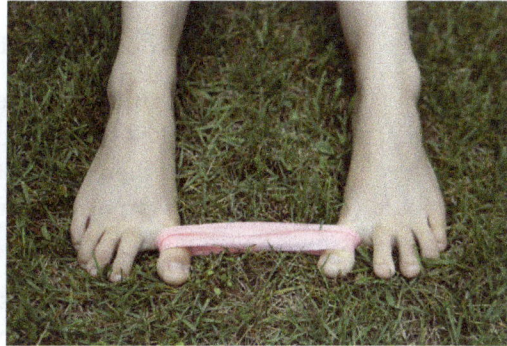

If you have a bunion already forming, some great ways to prevent it from getting worse is by stretching and strengthening.

- *Gently pull your big toe upward to stretch the bottom, and then gently push it down to stretch the top.*
- *Try picking up marbles with your toes. This will help with coordination as well as strengthening your toes.*
- *Walk on the beach barefoot! The sand will help relieve any pressure as well as spread your toes apart for a nice stretch.*

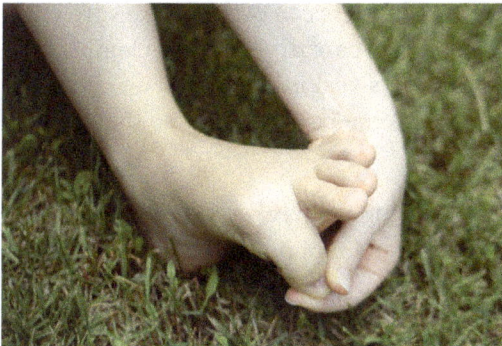
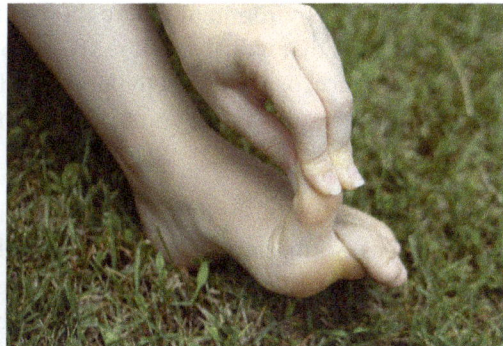

BLISTER PREVENTION

Blisters occur when there is constant rubbing of exposed skin and when there is excess moisture to that same area. The friction causes the layers of skin below the epidermal layer to tear. A clear liquid is then secreted to help protect the skin underneath. The liquid prevents infection and is there to help the skin heal faster. Because this liquid is so important to your healing, it is important that you do not pop your blisters. The best thing to do is to avoid blisters all together.

Make sure your dance shoes (and everyday shoes) fit well and form to your feet. If they are too loose, they can cause friction between the shoe and your foot creating blisters. You also do not want them to be too tight as the shoes can pull at your skin.

Every dancer has different spots on their feet where blisters tend to reappear, especially if you are *en pointe*. Protect your feet with toe tape, gel toe covers, or lamb's wool to keep your toes from rubbing against your shoes. When you take your shoes off after class, take notice of the red spots on your feet. Those spots are the ones that will most likely get a blister and need protecting the most.

When you dance, your feet sweat. There is no way to prevent it. If your feet are constantly in an environment where there is moisture, blisters can occur. Make sure you choose toe pads that will absorb the sweat so that your feet are dryer, such as lamb's wool, *Ouch Pouch*, or foam. Gel toe pads tend to trap the sweat inside. If you do choose to use gel, however, make sure you wash your feet in between performances so that they stay dry.

If you do develop a blister in the middle of class or during the week, make sure you have items such as Antibacterial ointment, blister bandages, and foot powder. *Dr. Scholl's blister Band-Aids* provide a thick covering over the blister to prevent it from popping during class. Blisters aren't always preventable, but it is a good idea to try and avoid getting blisters as much as possible.

TOENAIL AILMENTS

Bruised Toenails

Bruised toenails can be very painful and can last for weeks or even months. When you are *en pointe*, the toenail can shift on the nail bed which then results in bleeding under the nail.

You want to make sure you keep your toes clean to prevent infection or bacteria from breeding under the nail. If the bruise is bad enough, your toe nail can fall off leaving unprotected skin. Make sure you keep this delicate skin protected by using bandages and antibiotic ointment to prevent infection.

To prevent bruising, make sure you are using enough padding when *en pointe*. Your toes can also be more prone to bruising if your toenails are clipped too short or are left too long. Make sure you clip your toenails just enough to keep them from being pushed up toward the cuticle when *en pointe*.

Ingrown Toenails

Ingrown toenails occur when the nail starts to grow into the skin instead of over it. It can be very painful and become infected if not treated properly or on time. The skin around the toe can become red and swollen.

Dancers struggle with ingrown toenails, especially pointe dancers, because their feet are in tight shoes for long periods of time. The pressure on the big toe can often cause an ingrown toenail. Cutting your toenails too short is the most common reason why dancers develop ingrown toenails.

The best ways to prevent an ingrown toenail:
- *Never cut your toenails too short. Cut them with the shape of your toe, trying not to cut down the sides too much.*
- *Use toe spacers to keep your toes from rubbing against each other. Properly protect the ends of your toes to keep the nails from being bruised continually.*
- *Keep your feet clean, off and on pointe, to prevent any injection from becoming a problem.*

If you have already developed an ingrown toenail:
- *Soak your feet in a warm bath with Epsom salts for about 10 minutes to relieve some of the pain and to take down inflammation. Epsom salts have antiviral, antibacterial, and antifungal properties that will help your toes and feet heal more quickly.*
- *Clean the infected part of the toe with hydrogen peroxide. If the skin around the nail is swollen, red, or hot, you can release some of the pus by gently pressing. Make sure you clean it immediately afterward to prevent infection.*
- *If your toe is not infected, place a small bit of cotton under the nail. This will hurt, but will help in the long run to keep the nail from growing into the skin. Apply some antibiotic ointment and cover it with a bandage.*
- *You can also drop some oil of oregano (Oregenol) on it to help it heal faster. The oregano kills off the organisms that contribute to injection, bringing relief.*

Toenail Fungus

Having toenail fungus is very unattractive but not painful. The toenails can become yellowed and thick. It is contagious so try not to share nail clippers or toe pads with fellow dancers. Catch it early so it is easier to treat. If you find that it is becoming harder to clip your nails, you should start treating it as a fungus.

The best ways to prevent fungus:
- *Air out your pointe shoes and pads – the moisture can breed bacteria and cause fungus to grow.*
- *Keep your feet clean and dry.*
- *Try and minimize the trauma to your toes by properly protecting them.*

If you develop fungus:
- *Soak your feet in a warm bath for 30 minutes. Drop 10 drops of Tea Tree oil in the water. Tea Tree oil is a natural fungicide and antiseptic. You can also create a mixture of Tea Tree oil and olive oil to apply under a bandage.*
- *Drop oil of oregano (Oreganol) on the affected area twice a day and cover with a bandage. Oil of oregano has antiseptic, antibacterial, antiviral and antifungal properties.*
- *Soak your feet in a cool bath with equal parts water and apple cider vinegar for 15-20 minutes. Repeat two times a day.*
- *Soak your feet in equal parts water and hydrogen peroxide for 15-20 minutes.*

PROTECTING YOUR TOES EN POINTE

It is so important that dancers who are *en pointe* properly protect their feet while dancing. Use proper padding such as toe tape, toe wrap, pointe pads, toe separators, and lamb's wool. It is also important to have Band-Aids available for any injuries.

Proper padding and protection will help your feet in the long run. I recommend *Pillows for Pointe Gel Tip Toe Pillows*, *Ouch Pouch by Bunheads*, *Lamb's Wool by Freed of London*, *Bunheads Toe Tape*, and *Gaynor Minden Toe Wrap Foam Tape*.

A lot of dancers tend to put Advil gel on their toes in order to reduce pain from pointe shoes. Because your skin absorbs everything that is placed on the surface, you want to avoid using NSAIDs for pain. You will remember from chapter 2 that NSAIDs can cause long term health complications.

Instead of using the Advil gels, I recommend that you try a cayenne ointment. Cayenne contains capsaicin, which is an anti-inflammatory compound found in hot peppers. Try mixing 2 tablespoons of cayenne and ½ cup of coconut oil together in an air-tight container. Apply a little to your source of pain when needed.

PROPER SHOE CHOICES

Flip-Flops

Flip-Flops are usually what dancers choose to wear when they need to remove their shoes quickly. It is also very popular to wear them in the summer when you want your toes to breathe a little. The downsides to flip-flops, however, are many and might make you think twice before wearing them every day.

There have been links between flip-flops and tendonitis. The constant gripping of the toes tires out the tendons causing inflammation. In addition, they do not provide any support thus the arch can drop causing flat feet.

The next time you go shopping for flip-flops or sandals, make sure you choose ones with arch support and a heel strap built in to keep your toes and arches happy.

High Heels

If you are like me, high heels are your go-to choice for a fancy dinner, party, or event. High heels, however can cause problems with your calves, Achilles tendon, and toes. The constant position of being in 'relevé' can shorten your muscles and cause them to contract giving you less motion in your calves and feet. They can also cause a lot of stress and inhibit the mobility of your joints and your Achilles tendon.

When you shop for your high heels make sure they fit and are comfortable. Stacy Barrows, PT, at Century City Physical Therapy in Los Angeles says, *"One test is to stand on the floor in the shoes with your knees straight, not locked. Raise yourself on your toes so there's at least an inch of space under your heels. If you can't do that, the heels are too high and you shouldn't wear them."*

Between Classes

To give your feet a break between classes, sneakers or any stiff shoe are your best choice. They give your toes a break by allowing them to rest inside the shoe without gripping. Make sure your shoe of choice has an arch support to avoid flat feet. My favorite brands are *Airwalk*, *Dr. Scholl's*, and *Aerosoles*. Kidney shaped shoes are also great for maintaining the natural shape of the foot.

EXERCISES AND RELAXATION

When you are done with classes, your feet could use a little TLC. Here are some exercises that you can do to stretch them out and relax the muscles. There are also some great at-home "spa" treatments that you can treat your feet to after a tough day of rehearsals.

Exercises and Stretches

Put your feet flat on the floor. Lift your big toe up to stretch the tibialis posterior (arch). The idea is to keep all your other toes on the floor as you are doing this. Lower your toe back down to the floor with some tension. Repeat 10 times.

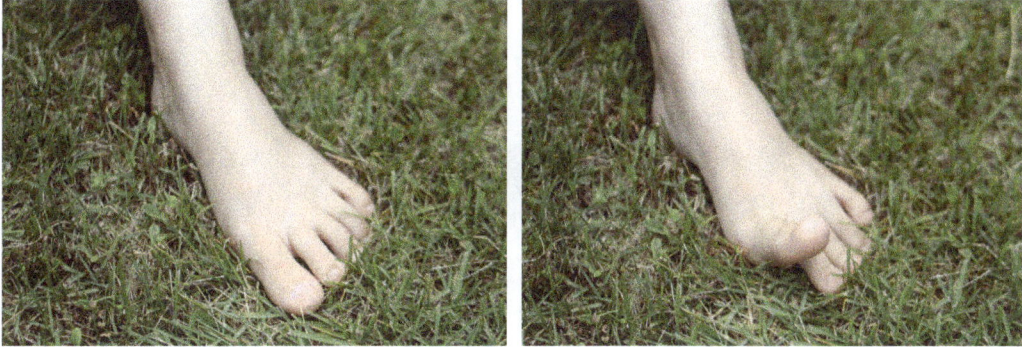

Place your hands on the wall for support. Put the balls of your feet on the wall, keeping your heel stationary on the floor. Bring your knee toward the wall slowly and hold for 30 seconds. Stop if you start to feel any pain. Perform 3 repetitions.

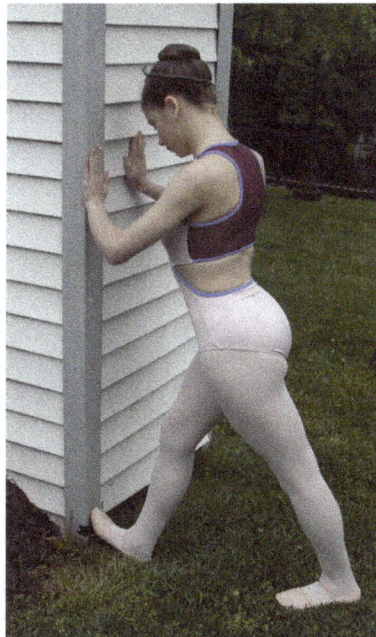

Tie a TheraBand around your ankle and around the barre. Raise onto half-pointe, keeping your knees in-line with your ankles. Repeat 20 times, making sure you are not rolling out.

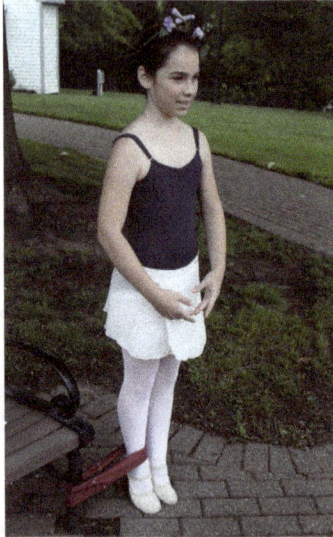

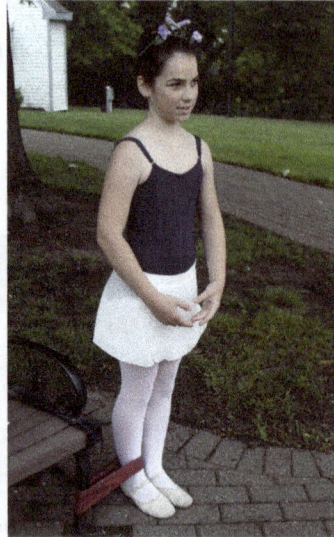

Start with your feet flat on the floor. Contract the arch, making a "bridge" with your feet and keeping your toes on the floor. This will strengthen the intrinsic muscles and prevent them from falling. Repeat 5-10 times.

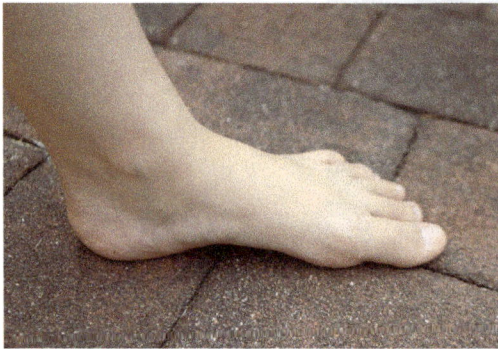

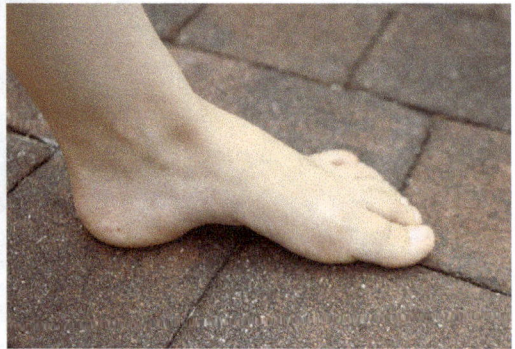

When you dance, it is easy to crunch your toes when you are trying to balance.

To practice keeping your toes stretched and relaxed while dancing, keep your feet flat on the floor, elongating your toes and creating space between all the metatarsals.

The muscle in the arch of your foot is called the tibialis posterior. It starts at the lower end of the calf and connects to the bone of the arch. When the muscle gets tired, the arch will drop.

To strengthen this muscle, you can perform standing calf raises. I recommend doing your calf raises on the edge of a step or block. Pull your heel toward the floor as you go down to allow a nice stretch in your calf before raising back up.

You can also perform calf raises with a tennis ball squeezed between your ankles. Make sure your ankles do not roll in or out as you raise up and slowly lower your heels back down to the floor. Repeat up to 20 times.

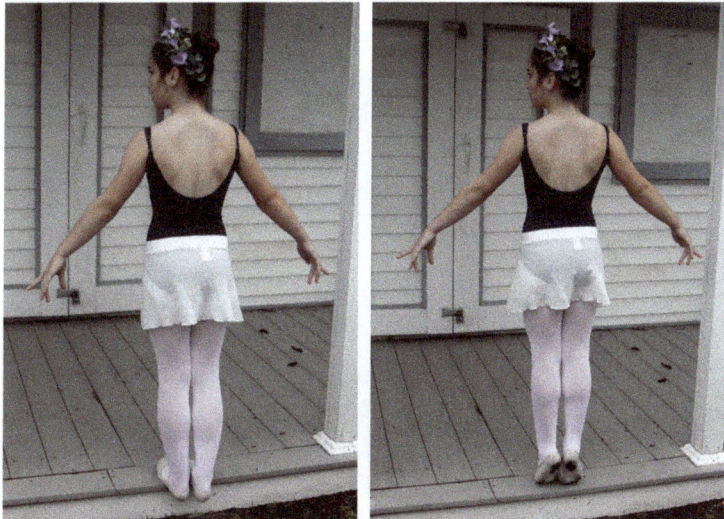

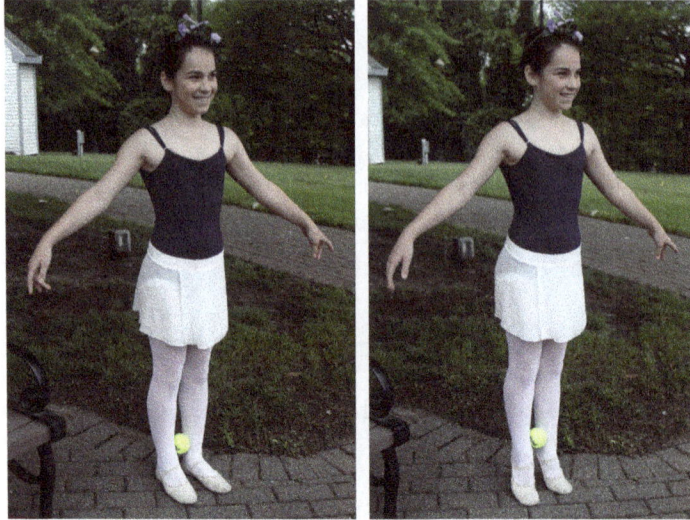

Walking barefoot is also very good for your feet. Walking on sand will allow your toes to spread, stretching them out and massaging the muscles.

Another way to stretch the tibialis posterior is to perform rotation or tension exercises.

Tension Exercises

Tie a TheraBand around the barre and wrap it around your foot. Sit on a chair parallel to the barre. Turn your toes inward creating tension in your ankle and arch. Repeat 10 times.

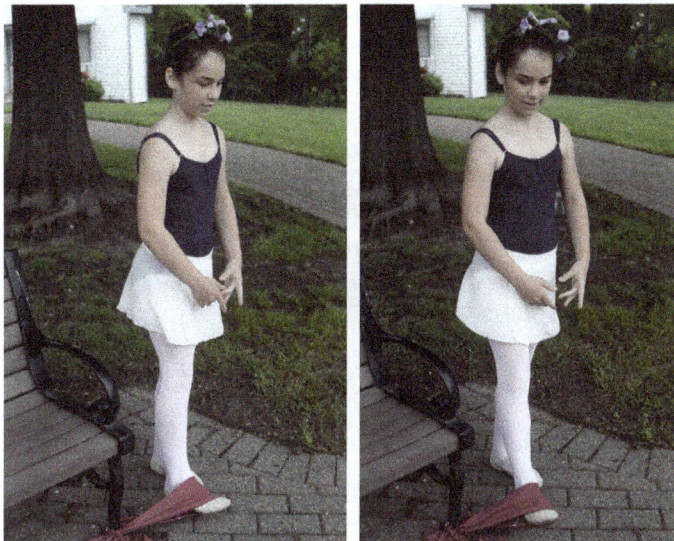

Clean your room with your feet! It sounds weird, but it is very effective. Instead of picking things up off the floor with your hands, do it with your feet. It strengthens your toe muscles and helps with your motor skills.

AT-HOME "SPA" FOR YOUR FEET

The constant jumping, pressure, stretching, and standing on your toes can make your feet look and feel very tired and sore. To rejuvenate your feet after a tough rehearsal, give them a warm bath.

Fill a tub or large bowl with warm to hot water. Drop about 10 drops of lavender (relaxation), peppermint (rejuvenation), orange or lemon (awakening) essential oil in the water. You can also add ½ cup of Epsom salts for detox.

Massage Techniques

Massage your feet to release the muscles. Use a body butter or massage oil and work from your heel to your toes. Don't forget to massage the top of your feet and your ankles, they need it too! To get the full effect, try these massaging techniques.

- *On the heel, use medium to heavy pressure with your thumbs. Move one thumb up and the other down. Repeat, always making sure you have one thumb up and the other down.*
- *Make circles around your ankles with your fingers.*
- *Use your knuckles to knead the arch. It tends to hold a lot of tension, so use heavy pressure – but be gentle.*
- *Massage in between each toe; then massage each pad of the toe with a medium to light pressure.*
- *On either side of the foot, use a pulling motion. Repeat ten times, alternating hands as you pull.*
- *Massage the balls of your feet with your thumbs using the same up-and-down motion as the heel massage.*
- *Massage the Achilles tendon and work up your calf, releasing any tension.*

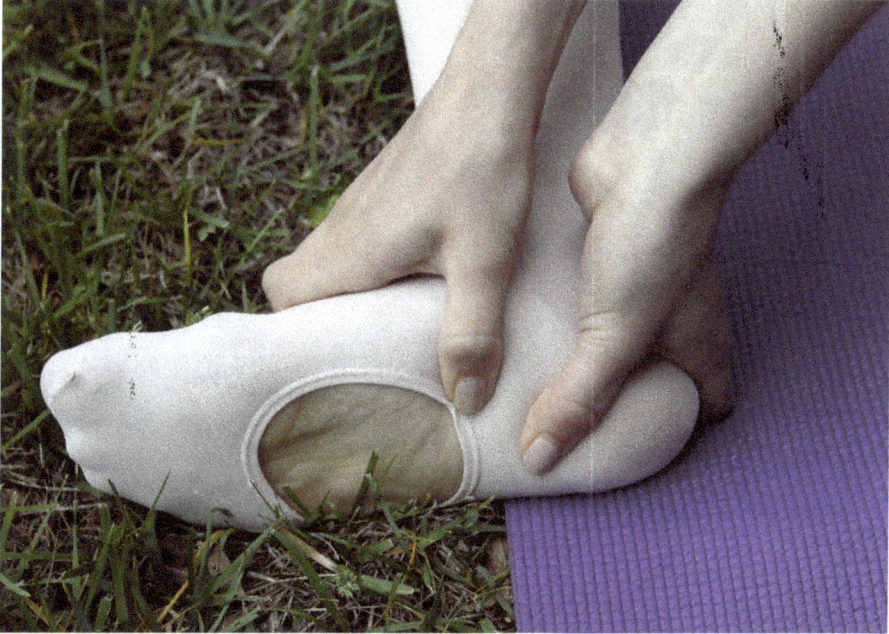

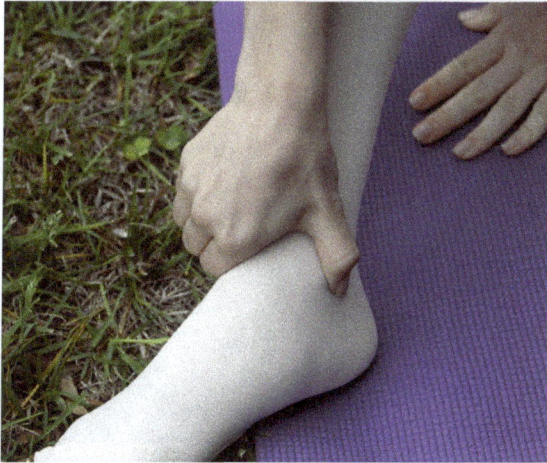
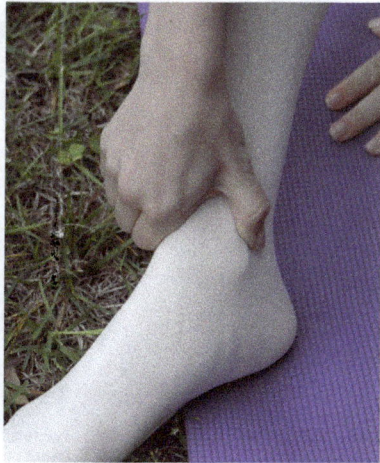

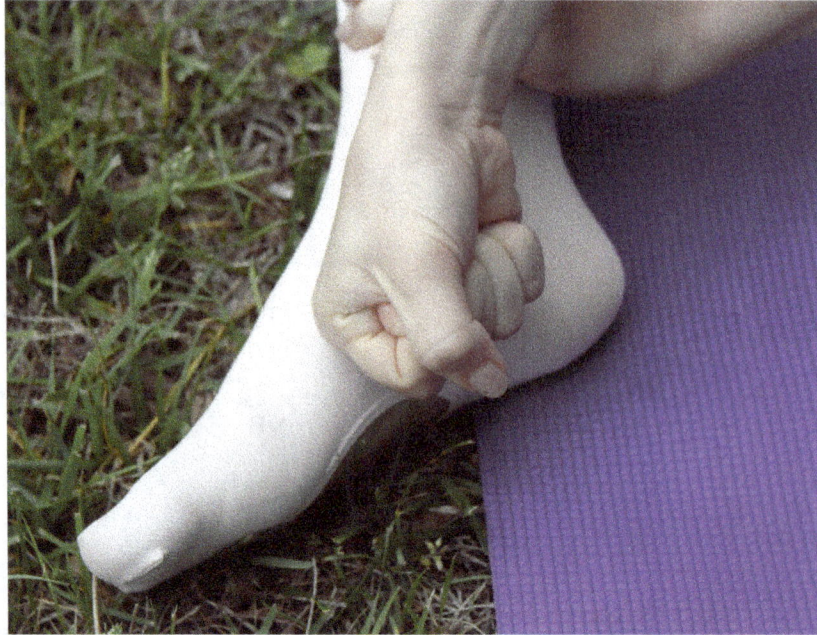

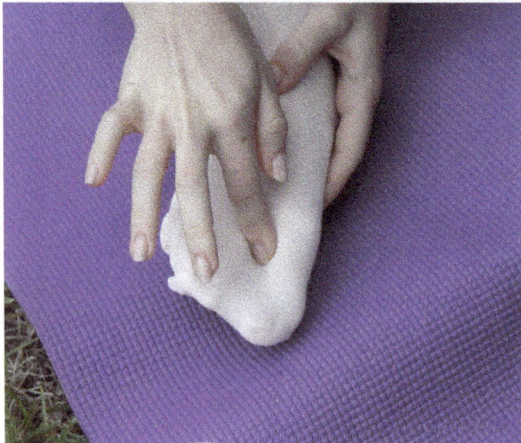

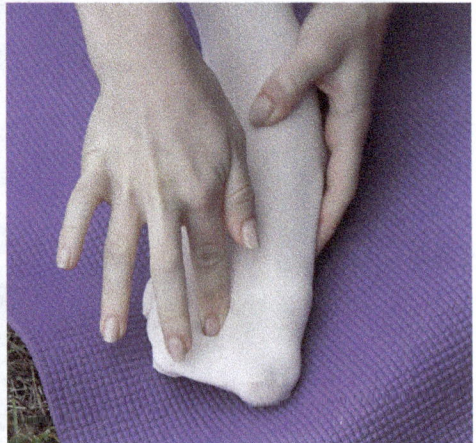

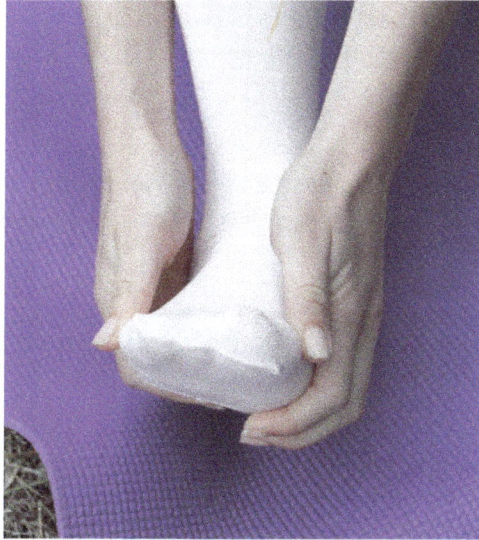
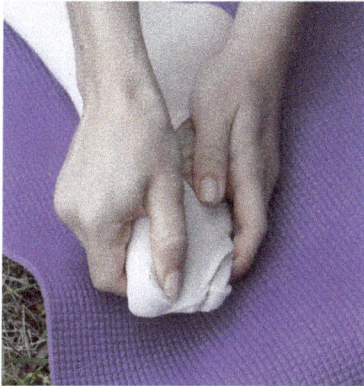
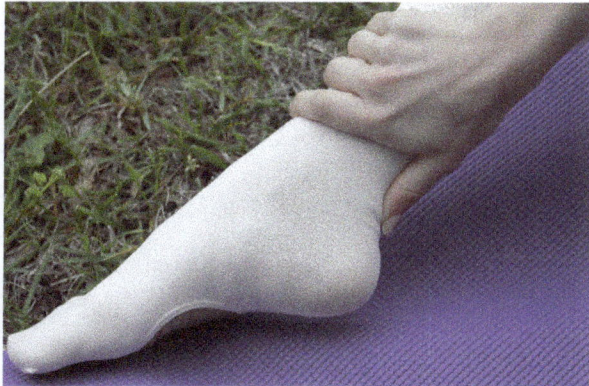
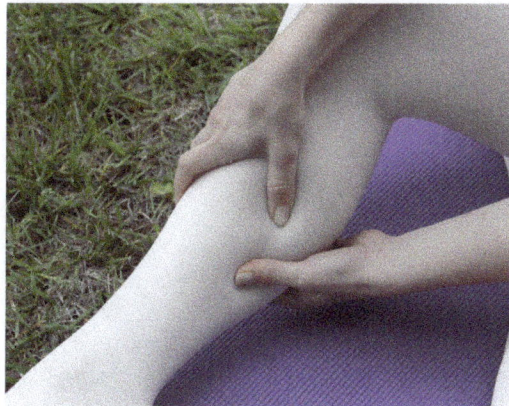

You can also use a soft ball or foam roller to massage and work out tight muscles if you do not have time to hand massage them. I recommend using a tennis ball or a *Surefoot Foot Rubz* ball.

If you are really sore, you can rub *Dr. Christopher's Complete Tissue & Bone* into your skin. It will penetrate deep to heal and soothe the muscles and bones. It is much more effective than any pain killer. It works best when applied twice a day especially after a tough day of rehearsals. Your feet will love you for it.

CHAPTER ELEVEN

Healthy Hair

Because of the constant need to have our hair in a bun while dancing, it can become broken and damaged. Thankfully, however, there are ways of repairing our hair with simple at-home remedies.

AFTER THE BIG PERFORMANCE

You have been under the bright lights, felt the tension and excitement, heard the roaring applause, and experienced the satisfaction of performing everything you have practiced since the beginning of the year. It seems all too wonderful for words, until you wake up the next morning and see all the damage that has been done to your lovely locks.

Split ends are extremely common among dancers. The constant pulling, brushing, and pinning breaks the ends leaving a frayed mess. One of the best ways to get rid of split ends is by having your hair trimmed every six to eight weeks.

In between the trims, however, make sure you are moisturizing your hair daily. Use a gentle conditioner when washing your hair, focusing on the ends. When you are not washing your hair, use other hair moisturizers such as *Moroccanoil*, olive oil, and coconut oil. The oils act as leave-in conditioners, and will bring luster and shine back into your hair. They are also great for keeping your hair strong and healthy.

Moroccanoil can be found in many different forms including, repairing masks, shampoos, treatments, styling creams, and conditioners. My favorite products include the *Moroccanoil Treatment Original, Weightless Hydrating Mask, Moisture Repair Shampoo and Conditioner, Smoothing Lotion, Frizz Control,* and *Heat Styling Protection.* These products can be found in most hair salons or online.

Coconut oil and olive oil are my favorite oils to use for damaged, dry hair. Coconut oil acts as a barrier, preventing water from being absorbed by the hair shaft. When water is absorbed into the hair, it can be more prone to breakage. Both oils also help with dandruff, make your hair shiny, and increase its manageability. Apply a small amount focusing on the very ends of your hair. You should purchase these oils in their purest forms, so look for extra virgin.

AT-HOME HAIR CARE

Sometimes it is nice to treat your hair to a "spa" treatment every once in a while. You can do most of the treatments in this section with items you can find around your home.

Try to limit your washing routine to every other day to prevent your hair from drying out. After a day of classes or rehearsals just rinse your hair and apply conditioner to the ends to remove excess oils and sweat. If you feel like you have to clean your hair, try using a natural dry shampoo.

Dry Shampoo

6-10 drops essential oil of your choice (EX: lavender, orange, eucalyptus, etc.)

2 Tbsp. cornstarch

2 Tbsp. rice flour

2 Tbsp. arrowroot powder

Mix together and sprinkle into your hair focusing on the roots.

If you have hair that tends to be oilier, add 1 tablespoon of lemon juice and half teaspoon of aloe Vera to your shampoo. The lemon removes the excess oils without stripping away the natural luster and shine and works in conjunction with the aloe Vera to improve hair growth. It also helps remove shampoo buildup on the scalp.

You can also try replacing your shampoo twice a week with a mixture of 1 Tbsp. of baking soda and 1 cup of water. Massage into wet hair avoiding the ends and rinse out with warm water. The baking soda will dry up excess oils on your scalp and will also help to remove any residue from the shampoo. Follow this with an apple cider vinegar treatment.

To prevent shampoo buildup, use apple cider vinegar 1-4 times a month instead of conditioner. Mix one part apple cider vinegar and one part water. After shampooing, pour the mixture in your hair and massage in. Let it sit for 5-10 minutes and rinse out with warm water until the smell is no longer noticeable.

For shinier hair add coffee grounds to your conditioner. You can also put Epsom salts in for volume and shine. Try to stay away from harmful parabens and chemicals as they can cause health problems and strip away your hair's natural oils and color.

Drink plenty of water! Our bodies are 60-80% water so it makes sense that we would need to continue to stay hydrated for our bodies to work properly. Water helps support vitamin absorption and assists in healthy hair growth. Your hair is actually one fourth water so in order to maintain healthy hair, you must drink plenty of water each day.

Brushing your hair too much can cause breakage. Make sure you have a good brush that does not catch your hair and pull it. I recommend using paddle hair brushes with wooden or bamboo rounded pins or natural soft bristled brushes.

Another way to prevent breakage is to let your hair air-dry. The heat from electric hair dryers or curling irons can cause breakage and can dry out your hair faster and make it look dull.

When you are putting your hair up, make sure you use elastics that do not have metal pieces that could get caught in your hair and break it. Try using U pins instead of bobby pins. They tend to be looser and are less likely to break your hair.

Have fun with these simple remedies and experiment with them to see what works best for your hair.

CHAPTER TWELVE

Beauty Is More Than Skin Deep

Your feet and hair are important, but let us not neglect your skin. Skin is the largest organ of your body and plays many important roles such as thermal regulation, protection, constant generation of new cells, and converting sunlight to vitamin D. Maintaining a proper skin care routine helps keep your skin healthy and beautiful.

But remember, you are beautiful no matter what. As important as it is to take care of your outward appearance, it is more important to care for and cultivate a beautiful heart. Whatever is in your heart will ultimately show itself in your attitude and outward beauty.

FACIAL CARE

Before you start a skin care routine, you need to assess what type of skin you have.

There are three skin types; *oily*, *dry*, and *balanced*. Most people have balanced skin, which means that their skin is sometimes oily but mostly dry. Once you know what type of skin you have, it will be easier for you to purchase products and put together a routine that is best suited to you.

Washing your face with cleanser is best done at night to wash off all your makeup and sunscreen from the day. In the morning, just splash your face with a little lukewarm water to remove any extra oil. Cleansing your face too often can cause your skin to dry out and become flaky.

Use lukewarm water when rinsing your face as hot or cold water can cause capillaries to burst. Remove any eye makeup gently with makeup remover or with coconut oil, remembering to not pull on the delicate skin around the eyes.

Depending on your skin type, exfoliating can be done either every day or only a couple of times per week. Exfoliants act as skin brighteners and work similarly to toners. If your skin tends to be dry, exfoliate only a couple of times per week. For oily skin, you can exfoliate every day to remove the excess oils.

Exfoliants with small crystals like table salt and sugar, are best because they will not tear at your skin. Larger crystals or nut shells will catch and cause small tears in your pores. I recommend that you make your own exfoliant at home and tailor it to your own skin type and preferences.

Moisturizing is probably the most important part of your facial care process. If your skin is too dry, it is more vulnerable to peeling, cracking, and flaking. I used to forgo my moisturizer in the summer because my skin was so oily. Unfortunately, I had more breakouts and my skin did not look as healthy. If you have oily skin, use a moisturizer that is lighter and does not contain any extra oils.

You also want to make sure you are not over moisturizing your face as it can clog your pores. Coconut, olive, sweet almond, and jojoba oils can be used as natural moisturizers, and some can act as toners.

Products I Recommend

Honest Beauty Company:

I love this company because their products are all natural and have worked amazingly for my skin. The *Refreshingly Clean Gel Cleanser* is perfect for combination skin and removes all your makeup in one wash. *Even Brighter Everyday Moisturizer* works great for oily skin because it is absorbed quickly and does not leave a sticky residue. You can purchase these products online at *honestbeauty.com*. They also offer bundles that include the cleanser, moisturizer, and sunscreen specific to your skin type.

Aveda:

My favorite products from Aveda are the *Outer Peace Foaming Cleanser* and the *Botanical Kinetics Exfoliant*. The exfoliant is great because it is a liquid that can be rubbed on the face with a cotton ball. It is gentle and you can start to see a difference within a couple days of using it. Your pores will get smaller and any acne will shrink overnight. These items can be purchased online at *aveda.com*.

Burt's Bees:

Burt's Bees has always been one of my favorite companies for natural care products. They offer a variety of products for all skin types including brighteners and anti-aging products. My favorites include, *Eye Makeup Remover Pads*, *Facial Cleansing Towelettes-Pink Grapefruit*, and *Garden Tomato Toner*. All these products can be found online at *burtsbees.com* and in select stores.

Yes To:

No matter what your skin type, Yes To offers products that cater to all using different fruits and vegetables that help tighten, exfoliate, and clean. Cucumbers are for sensitive skin, Tomatoes for combination and acne prone skin, Coconuts for dry skin, Grapefruit for uneven skin tone and dark spots, Blueberries for fine lines and wrinkles, and Carrots for normal to dry skin.

My favorites include *Yes To Tomatoes Daily Clarifying Cleanser*, *Yes To Grapefruit Brightening Facial Wipes*, and *Yes to Grapefruit Dark Spot Correcting Serum*. All products can be purchased in select stores and online at *yesto.com*.

Purchasing Beauty Products

When purchasing beauty products, avoid toxic chemicals such as parabens, synthetic colors, parfum, phthalates, triclosan, sodium lauryl sulfate, sodium laureth sulfate, formaldehyde, toluene, mineral oil, and propylene glycol. These additives can cause hormone disruptions and various health issues such as cancer, asthma, and skin irritation if used regularly.

When you use products with harmful additives, your skin actually absorbs them into the bloodstream. It is important that you choose products that are natural and organic such as ones I have recommended above. You can also make some of your own using the recipes I have provided below.

For oily skin:

Egg White Whip

1 egg white, whipped until stiff

1 Tbsp. lemon juice

Mix them together and apply to your face. Leave the mask on for 15 minutes and rinse it off with lukewarm water. Apply moisturizer immediately. The egg white will tighten the skin and absorb excess oils while the lemon balances your skin's pH and brightens dark spots.

Milk & Honey Mask

2 Tbsp. whole milk

1 Tbsp. honey

½ tsp. lemon juice

Stir all ingredients and apply in thin layer to your skin. Leave the it on for 10-15 minutes and rinse off with lukewarm water. Moisturize afterward. Honey is anti-bacterial and milk gently exfoliates and maintains natural pH in the skin.

Apple Cider Vinegar Toner

¼ cup distilled water

¼ cup apple cider vinegar

Shake both ingredients together in a bottle. Pour a little of the mixture on a cotton ball and wipe over skin. Moisturize as normal. Apple cider vinegar tones and moisturizes the skin as well as maintaining proper pH levels.

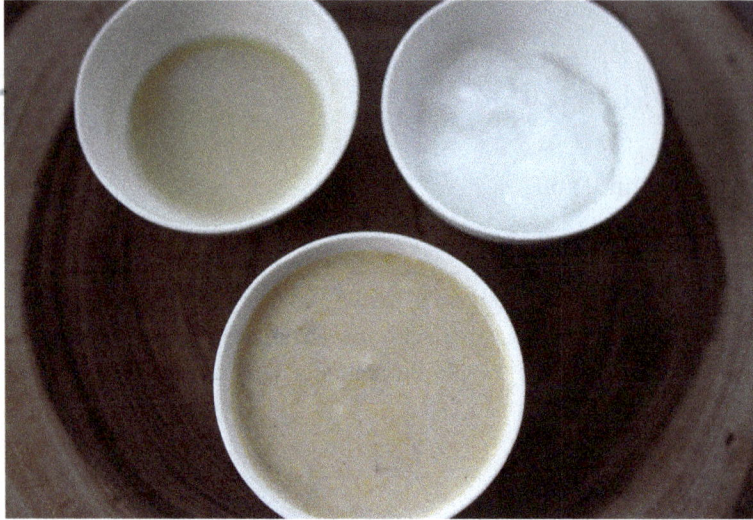

For dry skin:

Aloe Vera Cleanser

1 cup Aloe Vera gel

1 tsp. jojoba or coconut oil

8 drops grapefruit essential oil

8 drops sandalwood essential oil

4 drops rosemary or rosewood essential oil

Mix all ingredients together thoroughly. Massage into your skin using small, circular motions and rinse with lukewarm water. Moisturize immediately following. Aloe Vera soothes the skin and improves blood flow to the skin. The essential oil sandalwood, rosemary, and rosewood are anti-inflammatory and anti-bacterial.

Pumpkin Pie Mask

½ cup pumpkin purée

½ banana

¼ cup yogurt (Greek or whole milk)

1 tsp. cinnamon

Mash all ingredients together and apply to your face. Leave the mask on for 20 minutes and rinse it off with lukewarm water. Pumpkin increases collagen, protects against UV damage, and moisturizes the skin.

Avocado Face Mask

½ avocado

½ banana

2 Tbsp. yogurt (Greek or whole milk)

1 tsp coconut oil

Mash the avocado and banana together and then mix in the other ingredients. Apply to your skin and leave on for 30 minutes. Wash off with lukewarm water.

Other Recipes:

Dark Spot Reducer

½ tsp. baking soda

½ tsp. distilled water

Stir together and apply to dark spots. Leave this mix on for 5 minutes. Splash off with lukewarm water and dab hydrogen peroxide on with a cotton ball.

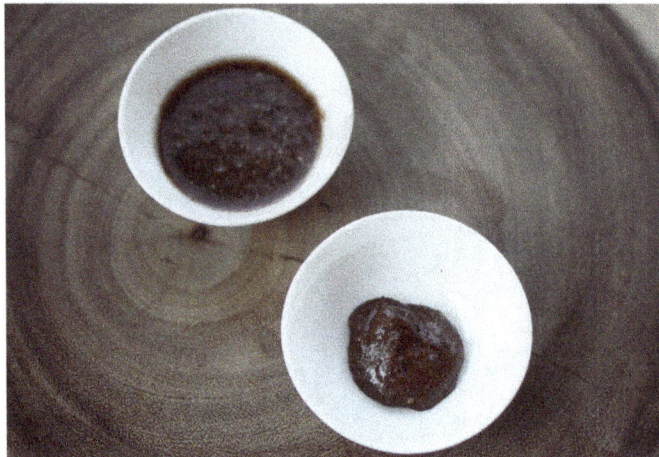

Spiced Exfoliant

½ tsp. honey

1 tbsp. coconut oil, warm

1 tsp. cinnamon

1 tsp. nutmeg

Mix together and gently rub in circles on your face. You can either wash it off right away or leave this mixture on for 30 minutes. Moisturize your skin afterward.

Sugar Exfoliant

1 tsp. coconut oil

½ tsp. brown sugar, or fine sugar

½ tsp. cinnamon

Mix everything together and gently rub into your skin, working in circles. Rinse it all off with lukewarm water and moisturize.

TIPS FOR HEALTHY, GLOWING SKIN

Your face is not the only skin that needs love and attention. Just with your face, your arms, legs, feet, and hands can use a little TLC sometimes to keep them silky smooth and glowing.

During dry months, make sure you are properly moisturizing your skin after you get out of the shower. The hot water tends to dry out your skin faster because all the natural oils have been washed away. Apply a small amount of natural lotion or body butter all over your arms, legs, feet, and hands.

Certain body products can cause pores to become clogged and inefficient at creating new skin cells. As with your facial care, make sure you are checking your body wash and soap for harmful chemicals that can be detrimental to your skin and health. The most common products that clog the pores are mineral oil, paraffin, and petrolatum. They can also show early signs of aging because they coat the skin, which builds up toxins on the surface.

Body scrubs can be used occasionally to remove dead skin cells and unclog pores, enhancing the natural "glow" of your skin. Gently rub the scrub in circular motions moving toward your heart and rinse off with warm water. Remember to choose a scrub that has small crystals so that you are not tearing at your delicate skin.

For cellulite:

Before you get in the shower, gently brush your skin using circular motions toward the heart. Dry skin brushing improves circulation and lymphatic flow, stimulates cell rejuvenation, and leaves your skin soft.

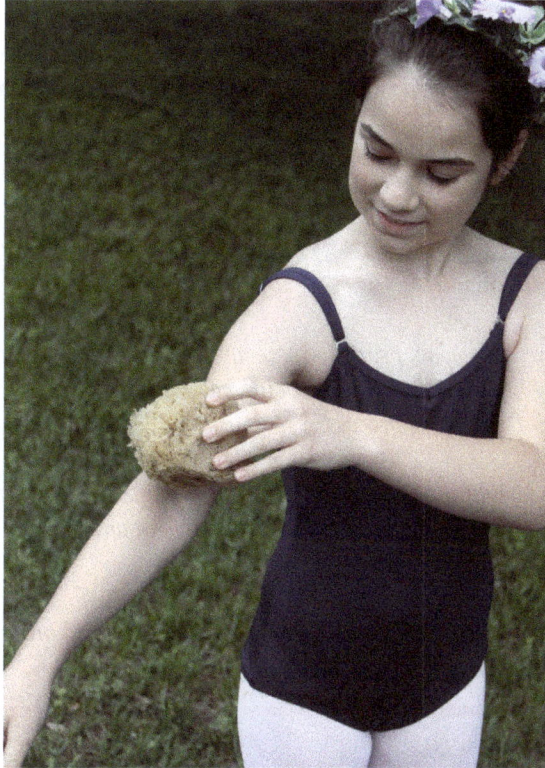

Cellulite Cream

½ cup coconut oil, melted

10-15 drops Juniper essential oil

½ teaspoon cinnamon

Stir all the ingredients together and pour into a jar. This mixture can keep for up to two months in a cool environment, completely sealed. Rub into your skin and leave on overnight.

Make a coffee scrub with equal amounts of ground coffee and coconut oil to rub into your skin. This can be applied after dry-brushing; rinse off. Coffee improves blood flow and coconut oil moisturizes.

For special skin conditions:

French green clay is great for acne, psoriasis, eczema and dermatitis. The clay is a mineral clay that is known for being highly absorbent, removing bacteria and infection. It is full of essential minerals that help with the healing process.

Make a mask by adding about a tablespoon of dry clay and just enough water or apple cider vinegar to make a paste. This mask can be applied 2-3 times a week and followed with moisturizer.

French green clay also helps remove excess lactic acid in overworked muscles. The mask can be applied to your muscles for relief.

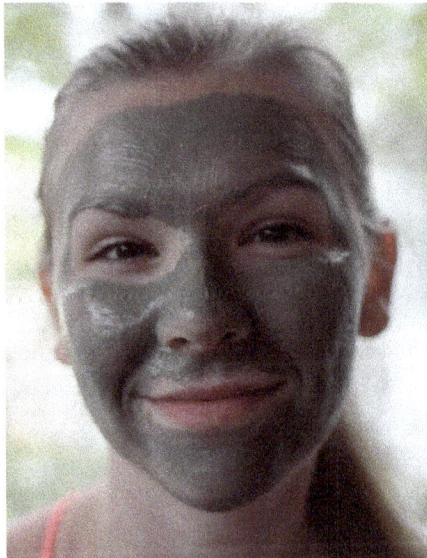

Even though these suggestions and recipes will help you achieve beautiful skin, maintaining a positive outlook on life and being peaceful is honestly the best way to stay healthy. Stress will cause breakouts because of the excess amounts of hormones released throughout the body. Stay calm and relaxed and do not be afraid.

"There's a difference between pretty and beautiful. When someone is pretty, they have a good appearance. But when someone is beautiful, they shine on the inside and out…"
   – Unknown

"Beauty is being the best possible version of yourself, inside and out."
   – Audrey Hepburn

"Beauty is about living your life and being happy with yourself inside and out, and not worrying about what people think of you."
   – Unknown

PART FIVE

Fun Stuff

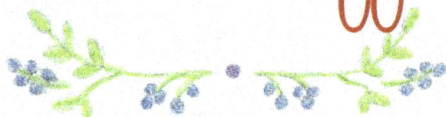

CHAPTER THIRTEEN

Additional Tidbits

DEVELOPING GOOD HABITS

All artists must practice constantly in order to master their chosen art. This takes lots of time and effort when it comes to achieving their goals. Dancers must learn how perform specific movements to music and this requires muscle memory. Gaining muscle memory, requires a lot of practice and discipline.

To create good habits, dancers need to focus on their ultimate goal and remember to not be too hard on themselves if they slip up. Learning from your mistakes is one of the best ways to continue excelling in your chosen art. Make sure that you are understanding what you are doing wrong so that you can fix it immediately. This way it does not turn into a bad habit.

Building bad technique can be detrimental to your dance career and can cause vulnerability to injury. Try to reverse it by learning it right and get help from your dance teacher and fellow students.

EVERYTHING A DANCER NEEDS TO CARRY WITH THEM

There are various items that a dancer should carry around in their dance bags. Having the right tools to perform is important for all artists. Depending on the level of dance you are in, I have listed all the items that you might need to carry in your dance bag.

Dancers who are just starting out or are not yet on pointe should carry items such as extra shoes, tights, and leotards, warm-up items (*sweaters, leg warmers, dancer shorts*), bobby pins and hair ties, hairspray, TheraBand, deodorant, hand sanitizer, and a mini emergency kit with items like arnica gel, band aids, ibuprofen, and antibacterial ointment.

Advanced and pointe dancers need to carry much more with them because of sore muscles and blisters. A small emergency kit is super important for pointe dancers. It can contain arnica gel, band aids, ace bandages, ibuprofen, antibacterial ointment, *Bunheads* muscle and joint gel, toe tape, second skin, oil of oregano (for infections), *Germ-a-CLENZ* for feet, cold compresses, and heat packs.

Other items that should be included are deodorant, a tennis ball, bobby pins and hair ties, hairspray, brush, extra shoes, tights, and leotards, a book for downtime, warm-up items (*sweaters, leg warmers, dancer shorts*), TheraBand, and a mini sewing kit.

Any additional items that might be useful include a body roller (*Manduka*), a dance journal for any ideas that might come up, lotion, chapstick, makeup, and *Green Ballerina* foot soak.

All dancers should always keep snacks in their bag such as a piece of fruit (*banana, apple, or pear*), an energy bar (*Larabar, Raw Revolution, Health Warrior, and Vega Vibrancy*), or a nut and seed mix (*almonds, pecans, walnuts, cashews, pumpkin seeds, chia seeds, and sunflower seeds*).

Mints or gum such as Spry or Peelu are also great for quick breath fresheners or a little sweat treat. These kinds of gum have xylitol instead of sugar which can help keep your blood sugar levels low.

The most important item that you must have in your dance bag is water. I always bring either one large water bottle or two regular ones. It is extremely important that you have more water than you might need than not enough.

The checklist I have provided below should help you make sure you have the appropriate items to prepare you for class.

I wish you the best in your dance career! Just remember, you are beautiful and worthy of love. Dance because it gives you joy. Do not let anyone discourage you. Be the best you can be and that will be enough. If you ever want to connect, visit adancersdiarybook.com and sign up for the member's area to connect with me and other dancers around the country. I hope you enjoyed *A Dancer's Diary*!

Beginner's Dance Bag Checklist
Extra dance shoes, tights, and leotards
Warm-up items (sweaters, leg warmers, dancer shorts)
Bobby pins and hair ties
Brush
Hairspray
Deodorant
TheraBand
Hand sanitizer
Arnica gel
Band aids
Ibuprofen
Antibacterial ointment
Dance journal (*optional*)
Lotion (*optional*)
Chapstick (*optional*)
Makeup (*optional*)
Snacks (fruit, energy bars, or nut and seed mix)
Mints or gum
Water

Advanced Dance Bag Checklist
Extra dance shoes, tights, and leotards
Warm-up items (sweaters, leg warmers, dancer shorts)
Bobby pins and hair ties
Brush
Hairspray
A book for downtime
Mini sewing kit
Deodorant
TheraBand
Hand sanitizer
Arnica gel
Band aids
Ace bandages
Ibuprofen
Antibacterial ointment
Muscle and joint gel (*optional*)
Toe tape
Second skin
Oil of oregano
Germ-a-CLENZ
Cold compress
Heat pack
Tennis ball
Body roller (*optional*)
Dance journal (*optional*)
Lotion (*optional*)
Chapstick (*optional*)
Makeup (*optional*)
Snacks (fruit, energy bars, or nut and seed mix)
Mints or gum
Water

SIMPLE ANATOMICAL TERMINOLOGY

(alphabetical order)

Term	Meaning
Abduction	Moving away from the middle of the body
Adduction	Moving toward the middle of the body
Anatomical position	The standard position of the body in the study of anatomy from which all directions and positions are derived. In it the body is assumed to be standing, the feet together, the arms to the side, and the head, eyes, and palms facing forward.
Anterior	Closer to the front of the body
Cardiovascular system	Heart, blood vessels, and blood
Cartilage	Flexible connective tissue found in joints as well as ears and nose
Catabolism	The breakdown of complex molecules in living organisms to form simpler ones, together with the release of energy; destructive metabolism
Circumduction	Moving in a circular motion
Endocrine system	Hormones, pituitary gland, thyroid, adrenal glands, pancreas, and gonads
Epidermis	Outer, protective layer of skin
Extension	Straightening of a part; increasing the angle between two parts
Fascia	A thin sheath of fibrous tissue enclosing a muscle or other organ
Fibrin	An insoluble protein formed from fibrinogen during the clotting of blood. It forms fibrous mesh that impedes the flow of blood
Flexion	Bending of a part; decreasing the angle between two parts
Gastrointestinal system	Mouth, esophagus, stomach, small and large intestines, pancreas, liver, and gallbladder

Homeostasis	The tendency toward a relatively stable equilibrium between interdependent elements, especially as maintained by physiological processes.
Hyponatremia	A lack of sodium in the blood caused by excessive sweating, persistent diarrhea, or overuse of diuretic drugs
Iliotibial band (IT band)	A fibrous reinforcement of the fascia on the lateral surface of the thigh, extending from the upper part of the hip to the knee
Integumentary system	Skin, hair, nails, and gland in skin
Lactic acid	A colorless syrupy organic acid formed in sour milk and produced in the muscle tissues during strenuous exercise
Lateral rotation	Rotation away from the midline of the body
Lymphatic system	Tonsils, spleen, thymus, lymph nodes, lymphatic vessels, and lymph fluid
Medial rotation	Rotation toward the midline of the body
Metabolism	The chemical processes that occur within a living organism to maintain life
Metatarsal	Bones in the foot
Nervous system	Brain, spinal cord, ganglia, nerves, and sensory organs
Posterior	Closer to the rear of the body
Prone	Laying face downward
Protraction	Moving a body part forward
Respiratory system	Nose, pharynx, larynx, trachea, bronchi, and lungs
Retraction	Moving a body part backward
Supine	Laying face upward
Synovial joints	A joint cavity line with synovial membrane and filled with synovial fluid; allows for the most movement

Tendon	A flexible but inelastic cord of strong fibrous collagen tissues attaching a muscle to a bone
Tibialis posterior	Tendon that connects the arch of the foot to the calf muscle (gastrocnemius)
Urinary system	Kidneys, ureters, bladder, and urethra

THE HUMAN BODY ILLUSTRATED

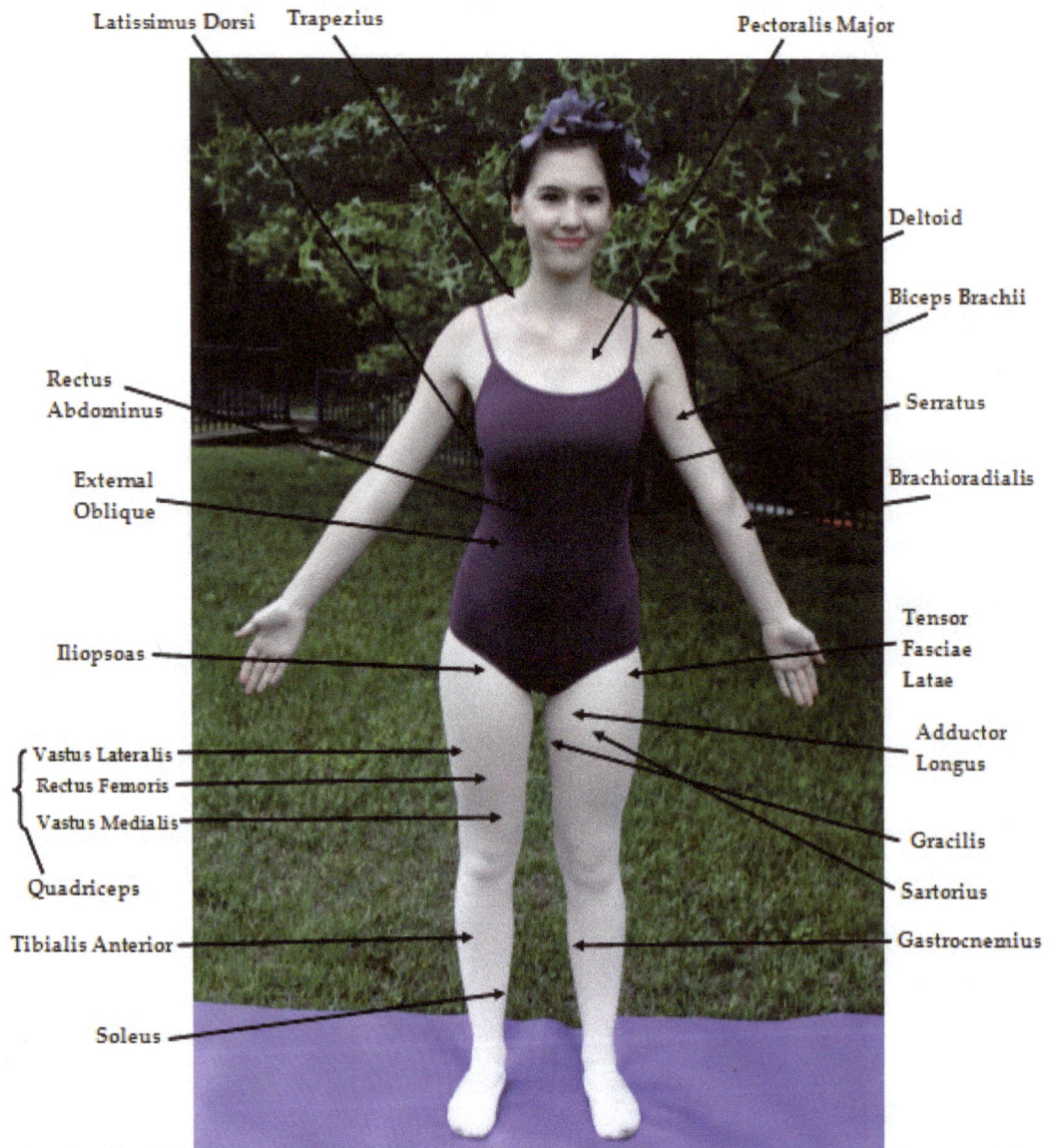

Latissimus Dorsi

Trapezius

Pectoralis Major

Deltoid

Biceps Brachii

Rectus Abdominus

Serratus

Brachioradialis

External Oblique

Iliopsoas

Tensor Fasciae Latae

Adductor Longus

Vastus Lateralis

Rectus Femoris

Vastus Medialis

Gracilis

Quadriceps

Sartorius

Tibialis Anterior

Gastrocnemius

Soleus

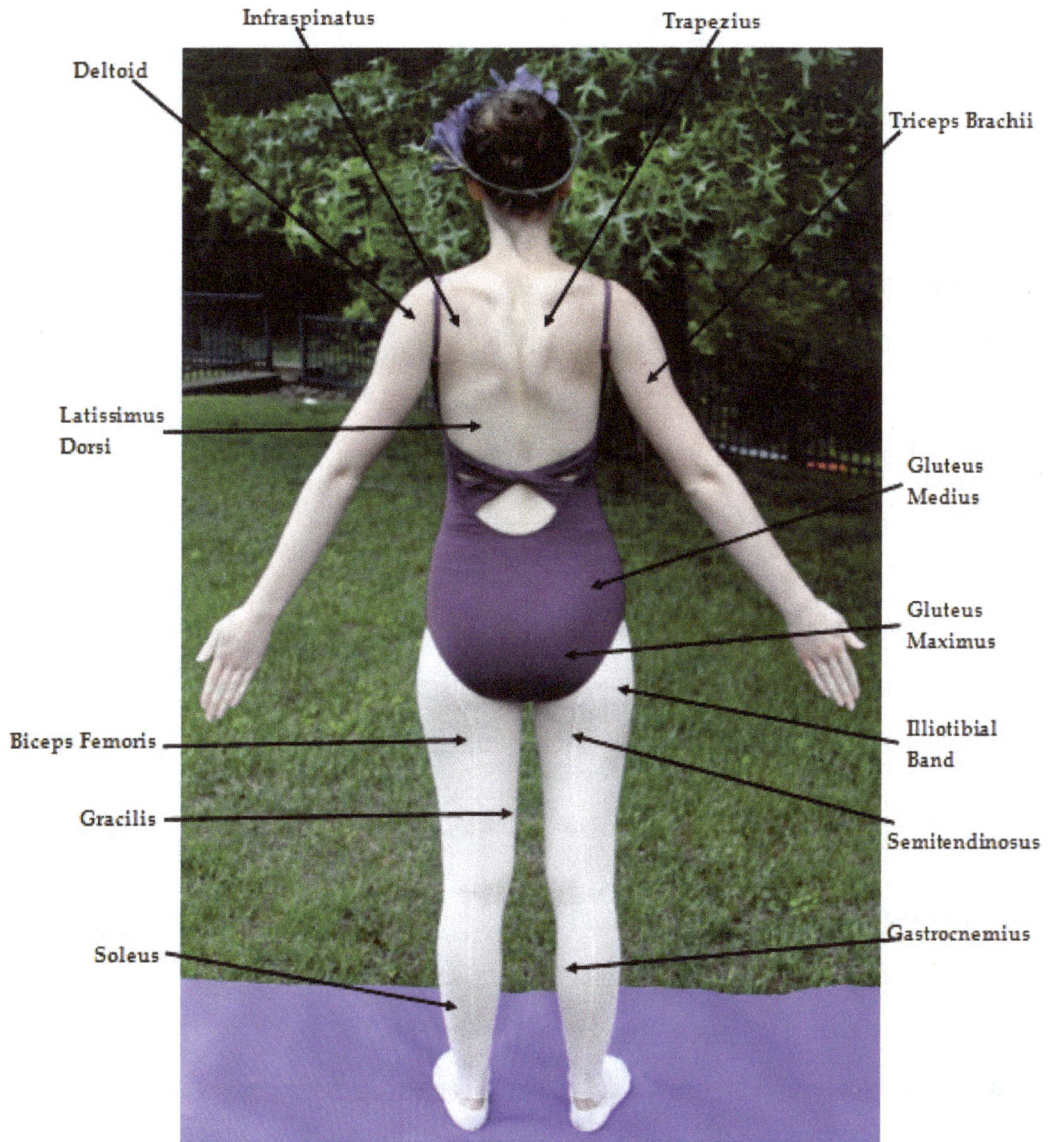

Deltoid

Infraspinatus

Trapezius

Triceps Brachii

Latissimus Dorsi

Gluteus Medius

Gluteus Maximus

Illiotibial Band

Biceps Femoris

Gracilis

Semitendinosus

Gastrocnemius

Soleus

Product Recommendations

A

ActivZ Coconut Water Powder (*activz.com, amazon.com, vitacost.com*)

Aerosoles Shoes (*aerosoles.com, amazon.com, JC Penney*)

Airborne (*airbornehealth.com, amazon.com, Walgreens*)

Airwalk Shoes (*airwalk.com, amazon.com, Payless*)

Allergy by Heel BHI (*vitacost.com, amazon.com, luckyvitamin.com*)

Almond Oil (*amazon.com, mountainroseherbs.com*)

Astragalus (*mountainroseherbs.com*)

Aveda Botanical Kinetics Exfoliant (*aveda.com*)

Aveda Outer Peace Foaming Cleanser (*aveda.com*)

Axe Nutrition's Vanilla Whey Protein (*store.draxe.com*)

B

Bergamot Essential Oil (*amazon.com*)

Berkey Water Bottles (*berkeywater.com*)

Brown Algae Extract (*amazon.com, luckyvitamin.com*)

Brown Cow Yogurt (*browncowfarm.com, Whole Foods*)

Bunheads Muscle and Joint Gel (*capezio.com, thedancewearshoppe.com*)

Bunheads Toe Tape (*capezio.com, discountdance.com*)

Burt's Bees Eye Makeup Remover Pads (*burtsbees.com, amazon.com, Target*)

Burt's Bees Facial Cleansing Towelettes — Pink Grapefruit (*burtsbees.com, amazon.com, Target*)

Burt's Bees Garden Tomato Toner (*burtsbees.com, amazon.com, Target*)

C

Calcium Lactate (*standardprocess.com*)

Chamomile Essential Oil (*amazon.com*)

Chestal (*chestal.com*, Walgreens, CVS)

Chicory (*mountainroseherbs.com*)

Collagen Protein (*store.draxe.com*)

Cumin Oil (*amazon.com*, Walmart)

Curcumin (*amazon.com*)

D

Daily Harvest (*daily-harvest.com*)

Dr. Christopher's Cayenne Pepper Extract (*drchristophersherbs.com*)

Dr. Christopher's Complete Tissue and Bone (*drchristophersherbs.com*)

Dr. Scholl's Blister Band-Aids (*amazon.com*, *drscholls.com*, Walgreens, CVS)

Dr. Scholl's (*drschollsshoes.com*, Walmart)

E

Echinacea (*mountainroseherbs.com*)

Elderberries (*mountainroseherbs.com*)

Epsom Salts (*amazon.com*, Target, Walmart)

Eucalyptus Essential Oil (*amazon.com*)

F

Foam Roller (*amazon.com*, Walmart, DICK'S Sporting Goods)

French Green Clay (*mountainroseherbs.com*)

G

Gaynor Minden Toe Wrap Foam Tape (*discountdance.com*, *allaboutdance.com*)

Gelsemium Sempervirens (*Walgreens*)

Germ-a-CLENZ (*amazon.com, vitacost.com*)

Ginseng (*mountainroseherbs.com*)

Grapefruit Essential Oil (*mountainroseherbs.com*)

Green Blender (*greenblender.com*)

Green Pasture Products Blue Ice Cod Liver Oil (*greenpasture.org, amazon.com*)

Green Ballerina Foot Soak (*greenballerina.com, amazon.com*)

H

Health Warrior Bars (*healthwarrior.com, vitacost.com, Whole Foods*)

Honest Beauty Company (*honestbeauty.com*)

I

Iceland Moss (*mountainroseherbs.com*)

Irish Moss (*mountainroseherbs.com*)

J

Jojoba Oil (*mountainroseherbs.com, amazon.com*)

L

La Croix (*lacroixwater.com, local grocery stores*)

Lamb's Wool by Freed of London (*freedoflondon.com, dancewearcorner.com*)

Larabar (*larabar.com, vitacost.com, amazon.com, Whole Foods*)

Lavender Essential Oil (*amazon.com*)

Lemon Essential Oil (*amazon.com*)

Ligaplex (*standardprocess.com*)

M

Maca Powder (*amazon.com, luckyvitamin.com*)

Manduka Body Roller (*manduka.com, amazon.com*)

Manuka Honey (*manukahoney.com, amazon.com, vitacost.com*)

Marcozymes (*pureformulas.com*)

MIT or TDP Lamp (*amazon.com*)

Moroccanoil (*moroccanoil.com, amazon.com, select Salons*)

N

Neprinol AFD (*amazon.com, neprinol.arthurandrew.com*)

Nettle Leaf (*mountainroseherbs.com*)

Nom Nom Paleo (*nomnompaleo.com*)

O

ONE Coconut Water (*onecoconutwater.com, Walmart, Target*)

Oreganol (*amazon.com, naturalhealthyconcepts.com*)

Oscillococcinum (*amazon.com, oscillo.com, Walgreens*)

Ouch Pouch by Bunheads (*capezio.com, dancewearsolutions.com, discountdance.com*)

P

Peelu Gum (*peelu.com, vitacost.com, Whole Foods*)

Peppermint (*mountainroseherbs.com*)

Perrier (*perrier.com, Walmart*)

Pillows for Pointe Gel Tip Toe Pillows (*pillowsforpointe.com, discountdance.com*)

Propolis (*amazon.com, luckyvitamin.com*)

R

Raw Revolution Bars (*rawrev.com, vitacost.com, amazon.com, Whole Foods*)

Rosemary Essential Oil (*amazon.com*)

S

Sage Essential Oil (*amazon.com*)

Serretia (*serretia.com, amazon.com*)

Smart Silver (*smartsilver.com*)

Spry Gum (*vitacost.com, amazon.com, Whole Foods*)

Sun Basket (*sunbasket.com*)

Surefoot Foot Rubz (*amazon.com, discountdance.com, footwearetc.com*)

T

Tangerine Essential Oil (*amazon.com*)

TheraBand (*thera-band.com, amazon.com, Walmart*)

Thyme Essential Oil (*amazon.com*)

V

Vega Vibrancy Bars (*myvega.com, amazon.com, livesuperfoods.com, Whole Foods*)

W

Wobenzym N (*amazon.com, vitacost.com, gardenoflife.com*)

Y

Yes To Grapefruits Brightening Facial Wipes (*yesto.com, amazon.com, Target, Walmart*)

Yes To Grapefruits Dark Spot Correcting Serum (*yesto.com, amazon.com, Target, Walmart*)

Yes To Tomatoes Daily Clarifying Cleanser (*yesto.com, amazon.com, Target, Walmart*)

Z

Zico Coconut Water (*zico.com, amazon.com, Walgreens, Target*)

Resources

A

Astaire, Fred Quotes. Imdb.com profile. 2012 – pg. 17:
https://www.imdb.com/name/nm0000001/bio?ref_=nm_ov_bio_sm

All About Water. "10 Reasons to Drink Water." 2012 – pg. 93-113:
http://www.allaboutwater.org/drink-water.html

Ahmed, Arshi. "22 Amazing Benefits of Water For Skin, Hair and Health." 2015 – pg. 93-113: http://www.stylecraze.com/articles/benefits-of-water-for-skin-hair-and-health/

Appleby, Maia. "Four Important Benefits of Carbohydrates." 2013 – pg. 93-113:
http://www.livestrong.com/article/504219-four-important-benefits-of-carbohydrates/

Antioxidants Detective. "The Benefits of Vitamin A." 2013 – pg. 93-113:
http://antioxidantsdetective.com/benefits-of-vitamin-a.html#.WS8A0IWcHIU

Axe, Josh DNM, DC, CNS. "9 Natural Ways to Treat Seasonal Allergy Symptoms." 2015 – pg. 134-140: https://draxe.com/seasonal-allergy-symptoms/#mobile-menu

Arthur Andrew. Neprinol Product Information. 2016 – pg. 38-60:
https://www.arthurandrew.com/products/neprinol

B

Brady, Krissy. "11 Benefits of Lemon Water You Didn't Know About." 2014 – pg. 93-113: http://www.lifehack.org/articles/lifestyle/11-benefits-lemon-water-you-didnt-know-about.html

Busch, Sandi. "Good & Bad Sugars." 2013 – pg. 93-113:
http://healthyeating.sfgate.com/good-bad-sugars-7608.html

Bishop, Kristin. "Keeping the Cold and Flu Away-Part 1." 2015 – pg. 134-140:
http://www.naturalnewsblogs.com/keeping-the-cold-and-flu-away-part-1/

Brian. "What is Tabata?" 2013 – pg. 21-34: http://tabataexercise.com/about-tabata-training/

Bush, Chelsea. "10 Signs You're Exercising Too Much." 2014 – pg. 21-34: http://health.usnews.com/health-news/blogs/on-fitness/2010/11/05/10-signs-youre-exercising-too-much

Big Knee Pain. "Water on the Knee." 2015 – pg. 38-60: http://www.bigkneepain.com/waterontheknee.html

Berry, Maryann. "3 Exercises to Improve Your Shoulder Mobility." 2017 – pg. 61-81: https://breakingmuscle.com/video/3-exercises-to-improve-your-shoulder-mobility

Bedinghaus, Treva. "Ingrown Toenail Treatment and Prevention." 2012 – pg. 171-187: https://www.thoughtco.com/ingrown-toenails-treatment-and-prevention-1006902

Brandt, Amy. "Oh, Toenail Woes!" 2012 – pg. 171-187: http://www.dance-teacher.com/oh-toenail-woes-2392442150.html

C

Charisse, Cyd Quotes. Imdb.com profile. 2012 – pg. 17: https://www.imdb.com/name/nm0001998/bio?ref_=nm_ov_bio_sm

Craig, Winston MPH, Ph.D., RD. "Health Benefits of Cumin." 2015 – pg. 38-60: https://vegetarian-nutrition.info/cumin-curry-and-cancer-protection/

Carter, Sherrie Bourg Psy.D. "The Tell Tale Signs of Burnout…Do You Have Them?" 2016 – pg. 150-155: https://www.psychologytoday.com/blog/high-octane-women/201311/the-tell-tale-signs-burnout-do-you-have-them

Cunningham, Vanessa. "10 Toxic Beauty Ingredients to Avoid." 2016 – pg. 189-200: http://www.huffingtonpost.com/vanessa-cunningham/dangerous-beauty-products_b_4168587.html

D

Daily Health Lifestyles. "20 Health Benefits of Coconut Oil." 2013 – pg. 83-92: http://dailyhealthlifestyles.com/20-health-benefits-of-coconut-oil/

Dance Magazine. "Your Body Tips 4." 2012 – pg. 93-113: http://www.dancemagazine.com/inside-dancemagazine/your-body-tips-4/

Dalleck, Lance C. Ph.D. and Weatherwax, M Ryan M.S. "Free Radicals, Antioxidants and Exercise: A New Perspective." 2016 – pg. 93-113:

https://www.acefitness.org/prosourcearticle/5688/free-radicals-antioxidants-and-exercise-a-new

Dorischua. "Natural and Home Remedies to Keep the Cold Away." 2015 – pg. 134-140: http://dorischua.com/2010/09/30/natural-and-home-remedies-to-keep-the-cold-away/

Drugs.com/Brightcom. "Sage." 2016 – pg. 38-60: https://www.drugs.com/npp/sage.html

Daily Natural Remedies. "10 Benefits of Turmeric." 2016 – pg. 38-60: http://dailynaturalremedies.com/10-benefits-of-turmeric/

Daily Natural Remedies. "10 Health Benefits of Ginger." 2016 – pg. 38-60: http://dailynaturalremedies.com/10-health-benefits-of-ginger/

Drugs.com/Brightcom. "What are Active Range of Motion Exercises." 2016 – pg. 61-81: https://www.drugs.com/cg/active-range-of-motion-exercises.html

F

FitDay. "How Much Exercise is too Much?" 2015 – pg. 21-34: http://www.fitday.com/fitness-articles/fitness/how-much-exercise-is-too-much.html

G

Garland, Judy Quote. Imdb.com profile. 2012 – pg. 17: https://www.imdb.com/name/nm0000023/bio?ref_=nm_ov_bio_sm

Gaynor, Mitzi Quote. Imdb.com profile. 2012 – pg. 17: https://www.imdb.com/name/nm0310989/bio?ref_=nm_ov_bio_sm

Griffin, Sharon E. B.S., M.S., Ph.D. "Soluble & Insoluble Fiber: What is the Difference?" 2014 – pg. 93-113: http://www.myfooddiary.com/resources/ask_the_expert/soluble_insoluble_fiber.asp

Get Healthy Life. "Bean Sprouts Health Benefits." 2014 – pg. 93-113: http://letsgohealthy.blogspot.com/2013/03/bean-sprouts-health-benefits-and.html

Gibson, Barbara. "Aerobic and Anaerobic Exercise: What is the Difference?" 2014 – pg. 21-34: http://www.fitness19.com/aerobic-and-anaerobic-exercise-what-is-the-difference/

Gangemi, Stephen Chiropractic Physician and Clinical Nutritionist. "NSAIDs-I Still Say Never." 2015 – pg. 38-60: http://sock-doc.com/nsaids_dangers/

Garden of Life. Wobenzym N Product Information. 2016 – pg. 38-60: https://www.gardenoflife.com/products-for-life-category/product-families/wobenzym-products

Gunnars, Kris BSc. "10 Proven Benefits of Green Tea." 2016 – pg. 38-60: https://authoritynutrition.com/top-10-evidence-based-health-benefits-of-green-tea/

Gonzalez, Kelly. "The Best Stretches to Avoid Injury in Your Favorite Sports." 2012 – pg. 171-187: http://www.livestrong.com/slideshow/1011403-stretches-exercises-outdoor-adventure/

H

HealthAliciousNess. "Top 10 Cholesterol Lowering Foods." 2012 – pg. 93-113: https://www.healthaliciousness.com/articles/foods-which-lower-cholesterol.php

Health Diaries. "7 Health Benefits of Vitamin C." 2014 – pg. 93-113: https://www.healthdiaries.com/eatthis/7-health-benefits-of-vitamin-c.html

Hayes, Hannah Maria. "Pain, Pain, Go Away." 2014 – pg. 38-60: http://www.dance-teacher.com/pain-pain-go-away-2392331851.html

Hanes, Tracii. "Natual NSAID Alternatives." 2015 – pg. 38-60: http://www.livestrong.com/article/110405-natural-nsaid-alternatives/

Ho, Wee Peng. "Top 10 Anti-Inflammatory Foods You've Got to Know." 2016 – pg. 38-60: https://theconsciouslife.com/top-10-anti-inflammatory-foods.htm

Heal With Food. "5 Health Benefits of Thyme." 2015 – pg. 38-60: http://www.healwithfood.org/health-benefits/thyme-healing-herb.php

Healing Histamine. "Thyme: Triple A Wonder Herb!" 2016 – pg. 38-60: https://healinghistamine.com/thyme-triple-a-wonder-herb/

Health Diaries. "10 Health Benefits of Broccoli." 2016 – pg. 38-60: https://www.healthdiaries.com/eatthis/10-health-benefits-of-broccoli.html

Homemade Medicine. "What Are Home Remedies?" 2016 – pg. 189-200: https://www.homemademedicine.com/

Hamlett, Shauntelle. "Health Benefits of Green Clay." 2016 – pg. 189-200: http://www.livestrong.com/article/233666-health-benefits-of-green-clay/

I

Inspiring Pretty. "15 Natural Beauty Recipes Using Everyday Foods." 2014 – pg. 186-188: http://inspiringpretty.com/2011/02/25/15-natural-beauty-recipes-using-everyday-foods/

J

Jarrett, Sara. "Eating to Boost Your Performance." 2014 – pg. 93-113: http://www.dance-teacher.com/celebrate-history-of-the-rockettes-2428017533.html

K

Kelly, Gene Quotes. Imdb.com profile. 2012 – pg. 17: https://www.imdb.com/name/nm0000037/bio?ref_=nm_ov_bio_sm

Karthik, Narayani. "Anaerobic Exercise Examples." 2013 – pg. 21-34: http://www.buzzle.com/articles/anaerobic-exercise-examples.html

Kaufman, Keith A. Ph.D. "Understanding Student-Athlete Burnout." 2016 – pg. 150-155: http://www.ncaa.org/health-and-safety/sport-science-institute/understanding-student-athlete-burnout

L

Live Science Staff. "30 Minutes of Exercise May Be As Good As 1 Hour." 2013 – pg. 83-92: http://www.livescience.com/22646-exercise-weight-loss.html

M

Mercola, Joseph M. DO. "A High-Fiber Diet Helps Boost Weight Loss." 2014 – pg. 83-92: http://articles.mercola.com/sites/articles/archive/2015/03/02/high-fiber-diet-weight-management.aspx

Mercola, Joseph M. DO. "More Evidence Adding Nuts Is a Healthy Choice." 2014 – pg. 83-92: http://articles.mercola.com/sites/articles/archive/2013/05/11/eating-nuts.aspx

Mercola, Joseph M. DO. "Artificial Sweeteners Gaining Increasingly Bad Press-and for Good Reason." Drs. Mehmet Oz and Mike Roizen 2014 – pg. 87: http://articles.mercola.com/sites/articles/archive/2013/10/23/aspartame-artificial-sweeteners.aspx

Mercola, Joseph M. DO. "What are the 10 Things That Can Pack on Pounds?" 2014 – pg. 83-92: http://articles.mercola.com/sites/articles/archive/2011/03/30/what-are-the-10-things-that-can-pack-on-pounds.aspx

Mercola, Joseph M. DO. "To Shed Pounds, You MUST Eliminate Fructose from What you Eat." 2013 – pg. 83-92: http://articles.mercola.com/sites/articles/archive/2011/07/29/foods-that-keep-you-thin.aspx

Mercola, Joseph M. DO. "10 Spices, Herbs That Aid Weight Loss." 2013 – pg. 83-92: http://articles.mercola.com/sites/articles/archive/2012/11/26/herbs-and-spices.aspx

Mercola, Joseph M. DO. "What You Need to Know About Vitamin K2, D and Calcium." Dr. Rheaume-Bleue 2015 – pg. 83-92: http://articles.mercola.com/sites/articles/archive/2012/12/16/vitamin-k2.aspx

Myers, Alexander Lee. "Are YOU Thirsty? The Perks of Dancers Staying Hydrated." Marie Scioscia, nutritionist-The Ailey School 2012 – pg. 93-113: https://sites.psu.edu/distresseddancer/2014/10/28/are-you-thirsty-the-perks-of-dancers-staying-hydrated/

Mercola, Joseph M. DO. "Vegetarian Move 'Forks Over Knives' Critically Reviewed." 2017 – pg. 93-113: http://articles.mercola.com/sites/articles/archive/2011/10/13/vegetarian-movie-forks-over-knives--critically-reviewed.aspx

Mercola, Joseph M. DO. "Certified 100% Organic Free-Range Chicken: An Exceptionally Clean, Healthy and Delicious Source of Essential Protein!" 2014 – pg. 93-113: http://products.mercola.com/organic-chicken/

Mercola, Joseph M. DO. "The Health Benefits of Fiber." 2014 – pg. 93-113: http://articles.mercola.com/sites/articles/archive/2013/11/25/9-fiber-health-benefits.aspx

Mack, Alicia Graf. Quote-Natural Health Magazine, Issue March/April 2014

MasterJohn, Christopher. "From Seafood to Sunshine: A New Understanding of Vitamin D Safety." 2013 – pg. 134-140: https://www.westonaprice.org/health-topics/abcs-of-nutrition/from-seafood-to-sunshine-a-new-understanding-of-vitamin-d-safety/#food

Mercola, Joseph M. DO. "Soy: This 'Miracle Health Food' Has Been Linked to Brain Damage and Breast Cancer." 2016 – pg. 134-140:

http://articles.mercola.com/sites/articles/archive/2010/09/18/soy-can-damage-your-health.aspx

Mercola, Joseph M. DO. "Tips for Surviving Spring Allergy Season." 2016 – pg. 134-140: http://articles.mercola.com/sites/articles/archive/2015/04/20/surviving-spring-allergies.aspx

Mercola, Joseph M. DO. "Anticholinergic Drugs: Studies Prove That These Drugs Make Your Brain Stop Working." 2015 – pg. 134-140: http://articles.mercola.com/sites/articles/archive/2010/08/03/tylenol-pm-causes-brain-damage.aspx

Mercola, Joseph M. DO. "One Early Morning Mistake (and 7 Others) You Don't Want to Make." 2013 – pg. 21-34: http://fitness.mercola.com/sites/fitness/archive/2012/04/20/interval-training-overcomes-workout-pitfalls.aspx

Mercola, Joseph M. DO. "Simple Prevention and Treatment Strategies for Back Pain." 2014 – pg. 21-34: http://fitness.mercola.com/sites/fitness/archive/2013/03/29/back-pain-treatment.aspx

Mercola, Joseph M. DO. "Static Stretching: How This Common Type of Stretching Can Damage Your Muscles and Tendons." 2014 – pg. 21-34: http://fitness.mercola.com/sites/fitness/archive/2013/03/15/improper-stretching-may-cause-injury.aspx

Mercola, Joseph M. DO. "Reasons Not to Stretch." 2014 – pg. 21-34: http://fitness.mercola.com/sites/fitness/archive/2013/04/19/pre-workout-stretching.aspx

Mercola, Joseph M. DO. "Extreme Endurance Exercise: If you Do This Type of Exercise, You Could Be Damaging Your Heart." 2014 – pg. 21-34: http://fitness.mercola.com/sites/fitness/archive/2013/08/23/extreme-endurance-exercise.aspx

Mercola, Joseph M. DO. "When and How Should You Warm up, Stretch, Exercise, and Cool Down?" 2015 – pg. 21-34: http://fitness.mercola.com/sites/fitness/archive/2010/09/08/when-and-how-should-you-warm-up-stretch-exercise-and-cool-down.aspx

Mercola, Joseph M. DO. "What Are Shiitake Mushrooms Good For?" 2016 – pg. 38-60: http://foodfacts.mercola.com/shiitake-mushrooms.html

Mercola, Joseph M. DO. "Sleep is Critical for Brain Detoxification, Groundbreaking Research Finds." 2016 – pg. 150-155: http://articles.mercola.com/sites/articles/archive/2013/10/31/sleep-brain-detoxification.aspx

Mercola, Joseph M. DO. "How to Use Coconut Oil for Hair Health." 2014 – pg. 186-188: http://articles.mercola.com/coconut-oil-for-hair.aspx

Mercola, Joseph M. DO. "The Ominus Truth Behind Cosmetic Beauty Claims…" 2016 – pg. 189-200: http://articles.mercola.com/sites/articles/archive/2010/08/14/red-alert-on-cosmetic-products-will-they-cause-a-health-disaster-like-asbestos-did.aspx

N

Nutrition and You. "Rosemary Herb Nutrition Facts." 2016 – pg. 38-60: http://www.nutrition-and-you.com/rosemary-herb.html

Nayyar, Namita. "Top 10 Health Benefits of Blueberries." 2016 – pg. 38-60: http://www.womenfitness.net/top10/blueberries/

National Sleep Foundation. "How Much Sleep Do We Really Need?" 2016 – pg. 150-155: https://sleepfoundation.org/how-sleep-works/how-much-sleep-do-we-really-need

Nail Fungus Home Treatment. "The Best in Home Remedies for Toenail Fungus." 2012 – pg. 171-187: http://www.treatnailfungus.org/home-remedies-for-toenail-fungus/

O

Olsen, Hanna Brooks. "Study Proves What You Already Knew: Sports Drinks Are Bad For You." 2013 – pg. 93-113: http://www.alloy.com/well-being/study-sports-drinks-are-bad-for-you-968/

Organic Facts. 2012-2016 – pg. 93-113: https://www.organicfacts.net/

Organic Facts. "11 Impressive Benefits of Sodium." 2013 – pg. 93-113: https://www.organicfacts.net/health-benefits/minerals/sodium.html

Organic Facts. "13 Incredible Potassium Benefits." 2013 – pg. 93-113: https://www.organicfacts.net/health-benefits/minerals/health-benefits-of-potassium.html

Organic Facts. "10 Amazing Benefits of Lemon Oil." 2015 – pg. 134-140: https://www.organicfacts.net/health-benefits/essential-oils/health-benefits-of-lemon-oil.html

Organic Facts. "11 Best Benefits of Bergamot Essential Oil." 2015 – pg. 134-140: https://www.organicfacts.net/health-benefits/essential-oils/health-benefits-of-bergamot-essential-oil.html

Organic Facts. "13 Best Benefits of Carrot Seed Essential Oil." 2015 – pg. 134-140: https://www.organicfacts.net/health-benefits/essential-oils/carrot-seed-essential-oil.html

OnHealth. Bursitis Injury. 2014 – pg. 38-60: http://www.onhealth.com/bursitis/page2.htm

Oxford Dictionary. Anatomical Terminology 2016 – pg. 206-208: https://en.oxforddictionaries.com/

P

Pittsburgh Ballet Theatre. "A Brief History of Dance." 2013 – pg. 18: https://www.pbt.org/learn-and-engage/resources-audience-members/ballet-101/brief-history-ballet/

Pou, Jackie. "The Dirty Dozen and Clean 15 of Produce." 2013 – pg. 93-113: http://www.pbs.org/wnet/need-to-know/health/the-dirty-dozen-and-clean-15-of-produce/616/

Pinel, Alexandra. "Wellness Sunday: Cross-Training For Dancers 101." Leigh Heflin MSC Dance Science 2013 – pg. 21-34: http://www.diydancer.com/cross-training-for-dancers-101/

Pure Formulas. Marcozyme Product Information. 2016 – pg. 38-60: https://www.pureformulas.com/marcozyme-250-tablets-by-marco-pharma.html

Physio Works. "What are the Benefits of Good Posture." 2016 – pg. 61-81: http://www.physioworks.com.au/FAQRetrieve.aspx?ID=31641

Q

Quinn, Elizabeth. "Too Much Exercise and Decreased Immunity." 2013 – pg. 83-92: https://www.verywell.com/exercise-and-immunity-3120439

R

Rogers, Ginger Quotes. Imdb.com profile. 2012 – pg. 17:
https://www.imdb.com/name/nm0001677/bio?ref_=nm_ov_bio_sm

S

Seattle Dance Circle. "A Brief History of Dance." 2013 – pg. 18:
http://www.seattledup.org/brief_history.htm

Schindler, LuAnn Quote. 2013 – pg. 19:
http://www.life123.com/sports/dance/ballet/history-of-ballet.shtml

Spector, Felicity. "Ballet Dancers: Under Pressure, and Underweight." 2013 – pg. 83-92:
https://www.channel4.com/news/ballet-dancers-under-pressure-and-underweight

Stewart, Kristen. "Does Muscle Weigh More Than Fat?" Pat F. Bass, III, MD, MPH 2014 –
pg. 83-92: http://www.everydayhealth.com/weight/busting-the-muscle-weighs-more-
than-fat-myth.aspx

Stahl, Jennifer. "Your Body Tips." 2012 – pg. 93-113:
http://www.dancemagazine.com/body-bits-2307026367.html;
http://www.dancemagazine.com/inside-dancemagazine/your-body-tips-2/

Sarah-The Health Home Economist. "The 9 Irrefutable Benefits of Cholesterol in the
Diet." 2014 – pg. 93-113: http://www.thehealthyhomeeconomist.com/the-9-benefits-of-
cholesterol-in-the-diet/

SFGate. "The Importance of the RDA." 2013 – pg. 93-113:
http://healthyeating.sfgate.com/importance-rda-3060.html

Sports MD. Injuries. 2014-2017 – pg. 38-60: http://www.sportsmd.com/sports-injuries/

SouthWest Nutraceuticals. Serretia Product Information. 2015 – pg. 38-60:
http://www.swnutra.com/store/p6/serrctia

Scott, Elizabeth MS. "How to Stay Healthy When You're Stressed Out." 2016 – pg. 150-
155: https://www.verywell.com/cortisol-and-stress-how-to-stay-healthy-3145080

Sorin, Fran. "13 Reasons Why Gardening is Good for Your Health." 2016 – pg. 150-155:
http://gardeninggonewild.com/?p=27941

Sagolla, Lisa Jo. "20 Essential Items to Pack in Your Dance Bag." 2016 – pg. 202-203: https://www.backstage.com/advice-for-actors/dancers/20-essential-items-to-pack-in-your-dance-bag/

T

The Funny Beaver. "30 Amazing Inspirational Quotes." Dan Coppersmith 2016 – pg. 131: http://thefunnybeaver.com/amazing-inspirational-quotes/

Teens Health. "How Much Sleep Do I Need." 2016 – pg. 150-155: http://kidshealth.org/en/teens/how-much-sleep.html

Top 10 Home Remedies. "Home Remedies for Oily Skin." 2016 – pg. 189-200: http://www.top10homeremedies.com/home-remedies/home-remedies-oily-skin.html/3

U

Urban, Shilo. "8 Reasons GMOs are Bad for You." 2014 – pg. 93-113: http://www.organicauthority.com/foodie-buzz/eight-reasons-gmos-are-bad-for-you.html

W

White, Dana Angelo. "Artificial Food Coloring: Good or Bad?" 2014 – pg. 93-113: http://blog.foodnetwork.com/healthyeats/2010/06/30/artificial-colors-are-they-safe/

Weening, Theo. "The Scoop on Grass-fed Beef." 2014 – pg. 93-113: http://www.wholefoodsmarket.com/blog/whole-story/scoop-grass-fed-beef

Wikipedia. "Aerobic Exercise." 2013 – pg. 21-34: https://en.wikipedia.org/wiki/Aerobic_exercise

Wozny, Nancy. "10 Common Dance Injuries." Michael Kelly Bruce 2015 – pg. 38-60: http://www.dance-teacher.com/10-common-dance-injuries-2392302154.html

Wozny, Nancy. "Your Body: Bad Step." Stacy Barrows, PT Quote 2012 – pg. 171-187: http://www.dancemagazine.com/your_body_bad_step-2306899215.html

WikiHow. "How to Give a Foot Massage." 2012 – pg. 171-187: http://www.wikihow.com/Give-a-Foot-Massage

Y

Yelhispressing Vibrations of a Heart: Historical & Romantic. Humor Quote by Paul E. McGhee, Ph.D. 2016 – pg. 150-155:
https://yelhispressing.wordpress.com/2015/11/06/laughter-2/

www.ingramcontent.com/pod-product-compliance
Lightning Source LLC
Chambersburg PA
CBHW080756300326
41914CB00055B/906